Clinical Epidemiology in Chronic Kidney Disease

Clinical Epidemiology in Chronic Kidney Disease

Guest Editors

Vincenzo Antonio Panuccio
Claudia Torino

MDPI

Basel • Beijing • Wuhan • Barcelona • Belgrade • Novi Sad • Cluj • Manchester

Guest Editors
Vincenzo Antonio Panuccio
GOM
"Bianchi-Melacrino-Morelli"
Reggio Calabria
Italy

Claudia Torino
Institute of Clinical
Physiology
National Research Council
Reggio Calabria
Italy

Editorial Office
MDPI AG
Grosspeteranlage 5
4052 Basel, Switzerland

This is a reprint of the Special Issue, published open access by the journal *Journal of Clinical Medicine* (ISSN 2077-0383), freely accessible at: https://www.mdpi.com/journal/jcm/special_issues/6LGUFG7Z2L.

For citation purposes, cite each article independently as indicated on the article page online and as indicated below:

Lastname, A.A.; Lastname, B.B. Article Title. *Journal Name* **Year**, *Volume Number*, Page Range.

ISBN 978-3-7258-7492-7 (Hbk)
ISBN 978-3-7258-7493-4 (PDF)
https://doi.org/10.3390/books978-3-7258-7493-4

Contents

About the Editors

Vincenzo Antonio Panuccio

Vincenzo Antonio Panuccio is a nephrologist and the Acting Director of the Nephrology and Kidney Transplant Unit in Reggio Calabria, Italy (since February 2025). He has been working in the same unit since 1991 and has served as an attending nephrologist since 1999. He graduated in Medicine from the University of Messina, Italy, and completed his specialization in Nephrology in 1997. He further trained at Erasmus University, Rotterdam, The Netherlands, with postgraduate certifications in Epidemiology and Data Analysis. His clinical and research activities focus on chronic kidney disease, dialysis, kidney transplantation, and hypertension. His main research interests include cardiovascular risk across different stages of chronic kidney disease, mineral and bone disorders, and quality of life. He is currently the principal investigator of two multicenter randomized clinical trials and has authored numerous publications in international peer-reviewed journals. He is also an Associate Researcher at the National Research Council, Institute of Clinical Physiology (CNR-IFC), Italy.

Claudia Torino

Claudia Torino earned a degree as a Doctor of Biological Science at the University of Messina in November 2002. After that, she received a PhD in the Pathology of Cell Proliferation and Differentiation (April 2009) and a Specialization Diploma in Clinical Pathology (October 2010) at the University of Messina. Presently, she is a researcher at the National Research Council, Institute of Clinical Physiology (CNR-IFC) of Reggio Calabria (Italy). Her areas of expertise are study design, prospective studies, case–control studies, cross-sectional studies, clinical trials, biostatistics, epidemiology, prognostic biomarkers, diagnostic biomarkers in chronic renal failure, and cardiovascular risk. She is a referent in the Bioinformatics Laboratory and a member of a Working Group working on "[drawing up] research protocols, submission to calls for tenders in the National and European sphere, [and] financial management of projects", both set up at the CNR-IFC. She is also responsible for monitoring the registries and clinical studies performed at CNR-IFC, Reggio Calabria, and is the Scientific Referent of National and International projects.

Journal of
Clinical Medicine

MDPI

Article

Impact of Serum Phosphate on Hemoglobin Level: A Longitudinal Analysis on a Large Cohort of Dialysis Patients

Vincenzo Calabrese [1,2], Giovanni Luigi Tripepi [3], Domenico Santoro [4], Valeria Cernaro [4], Vincenzo Antonio Panuccio [5], Sabrina Mezzatesta [3], Francesco Mattace-Raso [1,*], Claudia Torino [1,3] and on behalf of the Sicilian Registry of Nephrology, Dialysis and Transplantation [†]

1 Department of Internal Medicine, Erasmus MC, University Medical Center Rotterdam, 3015 GD Rotterdam, The Netherlands; v.calabrese@outlook.it (V.C.); claudia.torino@cnr.it (C.T.)
2 Department of Medicine and Surgery, University of Enna "Kore", 94100 Enna, Italy
3 National Research Council—Institute of Clinical Physiology, 89124 Reggio Calabria, Italy; gtripepi@ifc.cnr.it (G.L.T.); sabrinamezzatesta@cnr.it (S.M.)
4 Unit of Nephrology and Dialysis, Department of Clinical and Experimental Medicine, A.O.U. "G. Martino", University of Messina, 98122 Messina, Italy; dsantoro@unime.it (D.S.); vcernaro@unime.it (V.C.)
5 GOM "Bianchi Melacrino Morelli", Nephrology Unit, 89124 Reggio Calabria, Italy; enzopanuccio@gmail.com
* Correspondence: f.mattaceraso@erasmusmc.nl; Tel.: +31-(0)10-7035979
† Collaborators of the Sicilian Registry of Nephrology, Dialysis and Transplantation is provided in the Acknowledgements.

Abstract: Background/Objectives: Phosphate is a macro-element involved in all cellular energetic processes. As about 90% of the phosphate filtered by the glomerulus is excreted by kidneys, the impairment of renal function and the consequent over-secretion of parathyroid hormone and fibroblast growth factor 23 results in the increase in the serum phosphate levels. The association between phosphate and hemoglobin is controversial, as both direct and indirect relationships have been reported. The present study aims to investigate the relationship between phosphate and hemoglobin in a large prospective, longitudinal cohort including dialysis patients from the Sicilian Registry of Nephrology, Dialysis, and Transplantation. **Methods**: In this prospective cohort study, we included 6263 hemodialysis patients to achieve a total of 120,462 repeated measurements of serum phosphate and hemoglobin over time. The longitudinal association between phosphate and hemoglobin was analyzed by univariate and multivariate Linear Mixed Models. **Results:** The mean age was 66 ± 16 years and the median dialysis vintage was 5 months [IQR: 2–16]. Mean and median values of hemoglobin and phosphate were 10.7 g/dL (SD 1.3 g/dL) and 4.6 mg/dL [IQR 3.9–5.5 mg/dL], respectively. The multivariate model, adjusted for potential confounders, confirmed the positive association between serum phosphate and hemoglobin [adjβ = 0.13, 95%CI 0.03–0.23, p = 0.01)]. These results were confirmed in analyses stratified for the use of phosphate binders. **Conclusions:** In our large cohort of dialysis patients, we found a linear, direct relationship between phosphate and hemoglobin levels. As a reduction in phosphate is associated with a parallel reduction in hemoglobin levels, hypophosphatemia can accentuate anemia in dialysis patients. Our results generate the hypothesis that monitoring serum phosphate in clinical practice might provide a better management of anemia.

Keywords: dialysis; hemoglobin; FGF23; serum phosphate; longitudinal analysis

1. Introduction

Phosphate is a macro-element involved in all cellular energetic processes. Approximately 85% is deposited as crystals of hydroxyapatite in the bone, whereas the remaining 15% is stored in intracellular space as a component of nucleic acids and extracellular matrix [1]. About 90% of the phosphate filtered by the glomerulus is excreted by kidneys; thus, the reduction in nephron mass and the impairment of renal function are responsible for a reduction in phosphate excretion. As a consequence of this, from the early stages of chronic kidney disease (CKD) [2], parathyroid hormone (PTH) and fibroblast growth factor 23 (FGF-23), two hormones with phosphaturic activity, are over-secreted with the aim to regulate the serum concentration of this ion. Considering that dialysis patients are anuric, in this population, the over-secretion of the two hormones results in hyperphosphatemia, which, via FGF23, results in iron deficiency and anemia [3].

Although, in CKD patients, anemia is mainly caused by reduced erythropoietin levels [4–6], its onset has a multifactorial etiology. As proof of this, not only hyperphosphatemia but also hypophosphatemia impairs the hemoglobin level, suggesting a U-shaped association between phosphate and hemoglobin. Hypophosphatemia has been related to hemoglobin reduction both in experimental studies and in case reports. Low phosphate levels impair red blood cells' structure, with consequent hemolysis [7–10]. In addition, it reduces the stability of erythrocytes' membranes [11] and biconcavity [12] and increases hemoglobin oxygen affinity, which is in turn negatively related to hemoglobin concentration [13,14] Furthermore, hypophosphatemia increases phosphofructokinase activity and reduces ATP and the erythrocyte concentrations of glucose-6-phosphate and fructose-6-phosphate [15–18].

Due to the low prevalence of hypophosphatemia, current evidence mostly comes from case reports or case series, with only a small observational study (including 23 patients) and a case report involving uremic patients confirming this hypothesis [19,20]. Conversely, the impact of high serum phosphate on hemoglobin is much more studied, even though longitudinal studies are not available yet.

To our knowledge, no studies investigating the association between phosphate and hemoglobin and performed exclusively on dialysis patients have been published so far. More specifically, the association between serum phosphate and hemoglobin has never been longitudinally evaluated in dialysis patients.

The present study aims to investigate the possible association between repeated measurements of serum phosphate and hemoglobin levels in a large prospective cohort including dialysis patients from the Sicilian Registry of Nephrology, Dialysis, and Transplantation.

2. Materials and Methods

The study is in conformity with the guidelines of the Italian Data Protection Authority and in agreement with the Helsinki declaration. Ethical approval was not necessary based on the fact that the Sicilian Registry of Nephrology, Dialysis, and Transplantation [21] is a collection of regional data, instituted by regional laws. The Sicilian registry was created in 2008, with a decree (03423/08) that established its aim, i.e., collecting data and analyzing it. Informed consent is requested from all patients whose data are entered in the registry. However, as specified in art. 1, no formal approval from ethical committees is needed to analyze data as they are made available only in anonymous form.

2.1. Study Population Ad Laboratory Data

In this prospective cohort study, we included hemodialysis patients entered in the Sicilian Registry of Nephrology, Dialysis, and Transplantation from 1 January 2018 to 31 December 2020. Hemoglobin and phosphate measurements were collected from the start of the dialysis treatment. The median length of follow up was 52 [22–93] months. During this time, patients had a median number of 16 [6–39] measurements of hemoglobin and potassium.

Of the 6451 patients composing the original cohort, 101 were excluded because they were affected by hematologic disorders, and 87 were excluded because of missing serum phosphate and/or hemoglobin measurements, leaving 6263 hemodialysis patients, which facilitated a total of 120,462 repeated measurements of serum phosphate and hemoglobin over time (Figure 1).

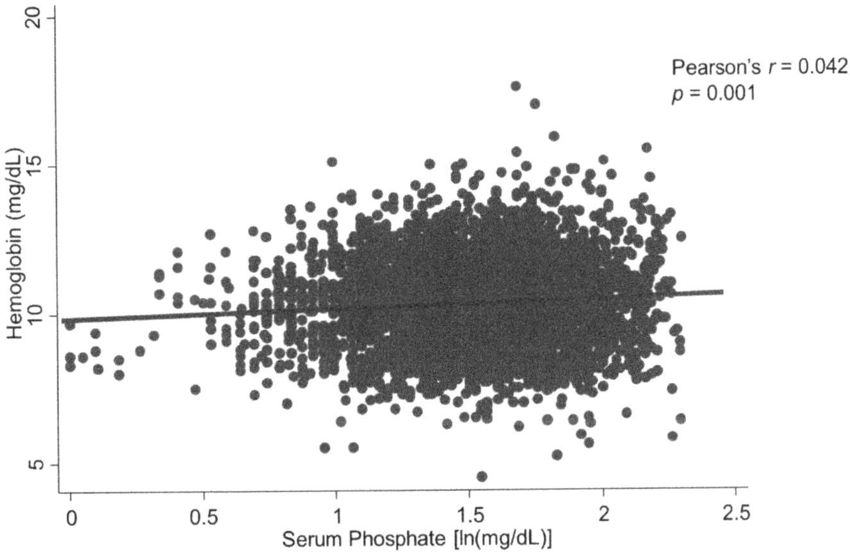

Figure 1. Scatterplot of the inter-relationship between serum phosphate and hemoglobin.

Patients had been on regular hemodialysis for a median time of 36 months (interquartile range: 10–78) and were being treated with standard bicarbonate dialysis with non-cellulosic membrane filters of various types (Enaxone, Elixone, Polyethersulfon, Polyacrylonitrile, Polyamide, Polymix, Polyethylene–Polyvin–Alcohol, Polymethylmethacrylate). In total, 3018 patients were treated with various anti-hypertensive drugs (874 on mono-therapy with ACE inhibitors, calcium channel blockers, α- and β-blockers, vasodilators, diuretics, or other drugs; 1033 on double therapy; 728 on triple therapy; and 383 patients on quadruple or quintuple therapy with various combinations of these drugs). The main demographic, somatometric, clinical, and biochemical characteristics of the study population are detailed in Table 1A,B.

Table 1. (**A**,**B**) Baseline characteristics of clinical, demographic, and laboratory data.

A	Whole Sample (n = 6263)
Hemoglobin (g/dL)	10.4 ± 1.3
Age (years)	66 ± 16
Sesso (male)	3904 (62.4%)
BMI (kg/m^2)	25.8 ± 5.1
DBP (mmHg)	72 ± 13
SBP (mmHg)	137 ± 19
Arterial hypertension (yes/no)	2366 (37.8%)
COPD (yes/no)	289 (4.6%)
Chronic liver disease (yes/no)	214 (3.4%)
Diabetes mellitus (yes/no)	1079 (17.2%)
Hemiplegia (yes/no)	32 (0.5%)
Heart failure (yes/no)	293 (4.7%)
IBD (yes/no)	54 (0.9%)

Table 1. *Cont.*

A	Whole Sample (n = 6263)
Malignancies (yes/no)	285 (4.6%)
Metastasis (yes/no)	57 (0.9%)
Vascular disease (yes/no)	262 (4.2%)
Albumin (g/dL)	3.58 ± 0.56
Cholesterol (mg/dL)	158 ± 45
CRP (mg/dL)	2.9 [0.9–6.6]
Ferritin (ng/mL)	148 [16–314]
Serum glucose (mg/dL)	119 ± 48
HCO_3 (mmol/L)	21.8 ± 3.1
KT/V	1.32 ± 0.33
iPTH (pg/mL)	228 [112–391]
Potassium (mmol/L)	4.9 ± 0.8
Triglycerides (mg/dL)	140 ± 79
Transferrin saturation (%)	23 ± 15
B	**Whole Sample (n = 6263)**
ACEI (yes/no)	460 (7.3%)
Folic acid (yes/no)	586 (9.4%)
Calcium carbonate (yes/no)	514 (8.2%)
Cholecalciferol (yes/no)	138 (2.2%)
Cortisone therapy (yes/no)	166 (2.7%)
Dementia (yes/no)	80 (1.3%)
Diuretic (yes/no)	1627 (26%)
ESA (yes/no)	2900 (46.3%)
Iron supplementation (yes/no)	0 (0%)
Immunosuppression (yes/no)	15 (0.2%)
PPI (yes/no)	2373 (37.9%)
Paricalcitol (yes/no)	486 (7.8%)
Sevelamer (yes/no)	1469 (23.5%)
Vitamin B12 (yes/no)	176 (2.8%)

BMI: body mass index; COPD: chronic obstructive pulmonary disease; IBD: inflammatory Bowel Diseases; DBP: diastolic blood pressure; iPTH: intact parathormone; CRP: C-reactive protein; SBP: systolic blood pressure. ACEI: angiotensin convertase enzyme inhibitor; ESA: erythropoietin-stimulating agent; PPI: protonic pump inhibitors.

2.2. Data Collection

Laboratory and clinical data were collected locally from the Register referents as part of the normal clinical practice and then entered in the platform. Laboratory data included serum phosphate, hemoglobin, C-reactive protein, iron, transferrin, ferritin, potassium, calcium, intact PTH, albumin, glucose, triglycerides, cholesterol, bicarbonate, alkaline phosphatase, fractional urea clearance (Kt/V), and β2-microglobulin. Clinical data included blood pressure levels, residual diuresis, previous comorbidities (dementia, hemiplegia, liver disease, history of arterial hypertension, vascular disease, chronic obstructive pulmonary disease (COPD) malignancy with/without metastasis, heart failure, psychiatric disease, dyslipidemia, prostatic hypertrophy) as well as pharmacological treatment such as antihypertensives, folic acid, calcium carbonate, cholecalciferol, insulin, aspirin, allopurinol, phosphorous binder, calcium-mimetics, cortisone, erythropoiesis-stimulating factors (ESA), iron supplementation, immunosuppressive treatment, proton pump inhibitors, paricalcitol, and vitamin B12. Details of the registry are described elsewhere [21].

2.3. Statistical Analysis

Data were described as mean ± standard deviation, median and interquartile range, or proportion, as appropriate. Hemoglobin and phosphate, as well as the quantitative confounders, were included in the analysis as continuous variables. The distribution of variables was investigated by the Kolmogorov–Smirnov test followed by graphic evaluation. The number of missing data varied across variables. In detail, albumin was missing in about of 50% of measures, potassium in 38%, calcium in 22%, BMI in 21%, PTH in 58%, ferritin in 58%, CRP 75%, HCO_3 74%, and systolic blood pressure in 12%. Other variables included in the multivariate models had less than 0.01% missing data. Missing values were related neither to the center which provided the data nor to specific characteristics of the patients, so were considered at random. As mixed effects models are well equipped to handle missing (at random) response data if estimated using likelihood methods, we did not impute or recover them.

Baseline hemoglobin was described in the whole sample and according to quartiles of serum phosphate and compared using ANOVA test and Bonferroni post hoc analysis. The first quartile included patients with serum phosphate lower than 3.9 mg/dL (n = 1597), the second quartile, patients with serum phosphate between 3.91 and 4.5 mg/dL (n = 1456), the third quartile, patients with serum phosphate between 4.51 and 5.5 mg/dL (n = 1522), and the fourth quartile, those with serum phosphate higher than 5.51 mg/dL (n = 1688). The baseline correlates of serum phosphate and hemoglobin were tested by Pearson's product moment correlation coefficient (Supplementary Table S1). The analysis was also performed after excluding potential outliers, detected by graphical evaluation and by the Grubbs method (double sides).

The longitudinal association between phosphate and hemoglobin was analyzed by univariate and multivariate Linear Mixed Models. In adjusted analyses, we included as potential confounders all variables related to serum phosphate and hemoglobin with p value < 0.2. As Pearson's r was neither constant, nor constantly modified, nor contiguously modified visit to visit, the unstructured matrix was applied in the analysis. Multivariate models adjusted for sex, serum potassium, calcium carbonate, folic acid, iron supplementation, erythropoietin-stimulating agents (ESAs), paricalcitol, immunosuppressors, calcitriol, heart failure, peripheral vascular disease, diabetes, chronic liver disease, visit, KT/V, BMI, iPTH, transferrin saturation, serum ferritin, C-reactive protein (CRP), serum bicarbonate, serum calcium, systolic blood pressure (SBP), age, phosphate binders, ACE inhibitors (AceI), proton pump inhibitors (PPIs), arterial hypertension history, vitamin B12, diuretics use, cinacalcet use, dementia, malignancies without presence of metastasis, and chronic obstructive pulmonary disease (COPD) were evaluated through the analysis of residuals; the Hosman sensitivity analysis was also performed.

A sensitivity analysis was performed, computing missing values by multiple imputation using random forest methods with five sets of decisions, three for each imputation step. Final linear mixed model was also computed in this imputed database.

In order to exclude confounding by indication, the same analyses were performed when dividing the study population according to the use of phosphate binders.

To investigate the longitudinal effect of modification by age on the link between serum phosphate and hemoglobin, we included the following in the Linear Mixed Models: serum phosphate, age, and their product (serum phosphate*age).

3. Results

3.1. Baseline Analysis

The clinical, demographic, and somatometric characteristics of the whole population are shown in Table 1A,B. The mean age was 66 ± 16 years, and the median dialysis vintage was 5 months [IQR: 2–16]. Hemoglobin had a normal distribution with a mean value of 10.7 g/dL (SD 1.3 g/dL). Serum phosphate ranged from 0.89 to 9.99 mg/dL, was not normally distributed, and its median value was 4.6 mg/dL [IQR 3.9–5.5 mg/dL]. At baseline, the serum phosphate concentration was normal (i.e., 3.5–4.5 mg/dL) in 1771 patients (28.28%), low (<3.5 mg/dL) in 1003 patients (16.01%), and high (>4.5 mg/dL) in 3489 patients (55.71%).

These splits based on phosphate quartiles did not suggest a U-shape relationship (10.3 ± 1.3 vs.10.4 ± 1.2 vs. 10.5 ± 1.3 vs. 10.4 ± 1.5); in addition, Bonferroni post hoc analysis showed significant differences between the first quartile and the others (p12 = 0.08, p13 = 0.001, p14 = 0.01), but other differences were not significant. Serum phosphate and hemoglobin levels were positively associated (r = 0.042, p = 0.001) (Figure 1), and both variables were related to albumin, serum calcium, dementia, diabetes, serum bicarbonate, kT/V, COPD, malignancy, phosphate binders, serum potassium, reactive c protein, and heart failure (all $p < 0.05$, Supplementary Table S1). No association was found between hemoglobin and age (r = −0.015, p = 0.247). A sensitivity analysis, performed excluding outliers in ferritin, confirmed the result.

3.2. Longitudinal Analysis

The univariate Linear Mixed Model for repeated measures showed a direct association between serum phosphate and hemoglobin [β = 0.39, 95%CI 0.36–0.41, $p < 0.001$]. These results show that for each unitary increase in log-transformed serum phosphate, there was an augmentation of 0.39 g/dL on hemoglobin values or, in other words, for each unitary reduction in log-transformed serum phosphate, hemoglobin values were reduced by 0.39 g/dL.

The multivariate model, adjusted for potential confounders, confirmed the positive association between serum phosphate and hemoglobin [adjβ = 0.14, 95%CI 0.04–0.24, p = 0.01)] (Supplementary Table S2). In more detail, ESA, serum ferritin, serum bicarbonate, and systolic pressure were inversely associated with hemoglobin, whereas the other variables included in the model showed a positive association (Supplementary Table S2). The association between phosphate and hemoglobin was confirmed in the Hosman sensitivity analysis [adjβ for each unitary increase in phosphate = 0.16, 95%CI 0.06/0.26, p = 0.001] (Supplementary Table S3).

The same model computed in the imputed model did not significantly differ from the previous multivariate model, showing same direction and same significance of the association (Adjβ = 0.38, 95%CI 0.35/0.41, $p < 0.001$).

No interaction was observed between serum phosphate and number of visit.

As EPO and phosphate binders were prescribed according to hemoglobin and serum phosphate values, we considered them as potential sources of confounding by indication. For this reason, we performed a sensitivity analysis excluding these variables. Our results showed that additional adjustment or stratification for the use of phosphate binders did not change the results (Figure 2).

Figure 3 shows the association between phosphate and hemoglobin across age strata. In spite of the trend observed, which seems to suggest that this association was significant only in the age groups from 62 to 77 years, no effect modification by age (expressed as deciles) was observed (p = 0.19).

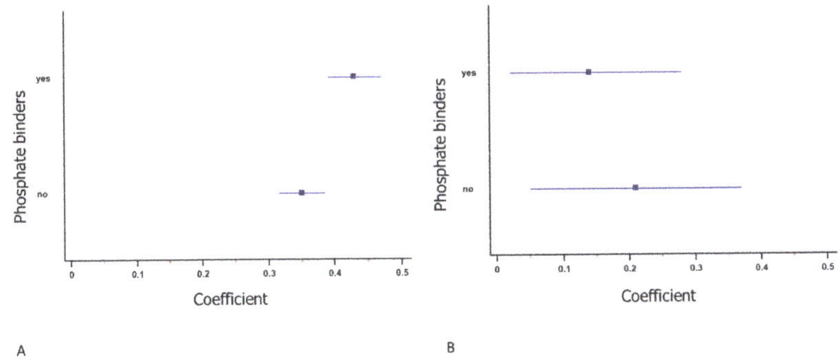

Figure 2. Forest plot of the association between serum phosphate and hemoglobin for patients who took phosphate binders. Both of them were positively related to hemoglobin both in univariate (**A**) and multivariate (**B**) analysis. The square represents the coefficient, and the line represents the 95% confidence interval. Upper lines show the coefficients in patients who assumed phosphorous binders, whereas lower lines show the coefficients in patients who did not assume phosphorous binders.

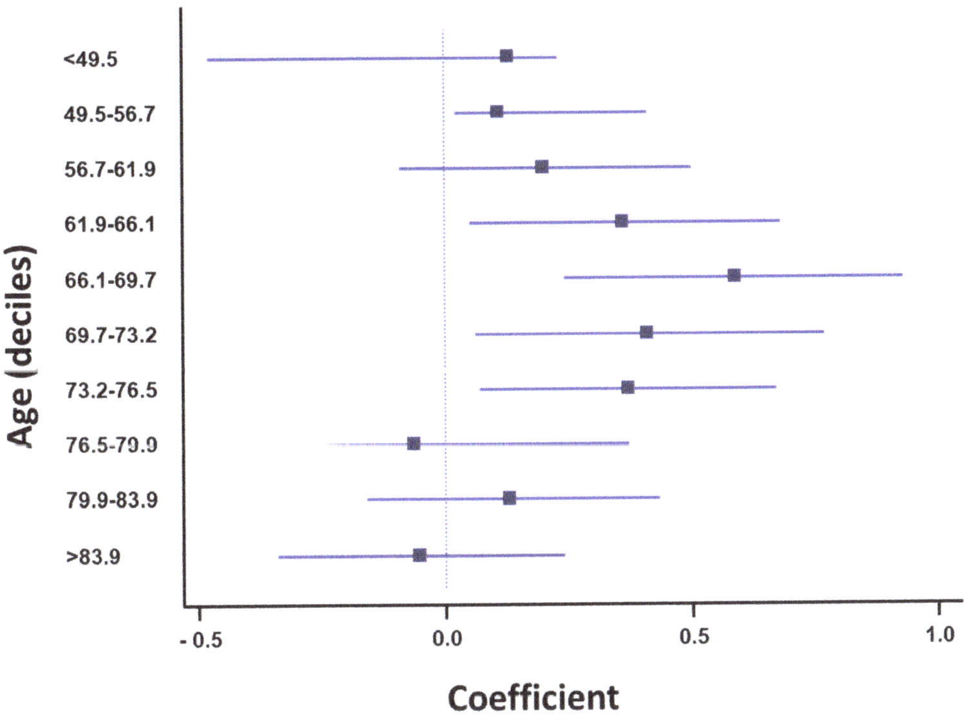

Figure 3. Forest plot of the association between serum phosphate and hemoglobin, stratified for deciles of age. Although no linear interaction was found, a trend was found in four deciles from 62 to 76.5 years. The square represents the coefficient, and the line represents the 95% confidence interval.

4. Discussion

In the present study, we found that, in a large cohort of dialysis patients, an increase in serum phosphate was associated with high levels of hemoglobin. Such an effect is independent from comorbidities, dialysis performance, therapy, and age.

As extensively reported in the literature, hemoglobin concentration is impaired both in hypophosphatemia and hyperphosphatemia [2].

Several mechanisms are involved in hypo- or hypophosphatemia-driven anemia. Hypophosphatemia is responsible for the reduction in ATP and 2,3-diphosphoglycerate levels, which in turn decreases the stability of the erythrocyte membrane through two mechanisms: the outward inhibition of calcium and structural damage. Low erythrocyte ATP impairs the calcium pump activities and inhibits the outward calcium flow. The excess of calcium binds to spectrin, thus damaging the membrane with consequent hemolysis [9]. Furthermore, ATP plays an important role in erythrocytes' biconcavity, so its reduction makes their structure unstable. As a direct consequence, the additional damages to the membrane and the alterations in the shape and size of erythrocytes, incompatible with the capillary flow, improves the risk of hemolysis, with consequent anemia.

On the other hand, hyperphosphatemia impairs hemoglobin levels via the overproduction of FGF23, in turn associated with iron deficiency [22,23]. High phosphate levels induce FGF23 overproduction as a compensatory mechanism, probably in response to PTH overproduction. FGF23 overproduction induces liver overstimulation of inflammatory molecules which impair erythropoiesis, reduce EPO excretion from the kidney, and block the erythrocyte cell cycle in G2, i.e., prevent them from completing the mitosis process [4,6]. Indeed, through hepatic pro-inflammation molecule secretion, FGF23 promotes hepcidin synthesis, reducing iron availability. In addition to the FGF23-mediated pathway, high phosphate levels may directly impair the hemoglobin level through toxic products such as the fetuin A [24].

Our analysis showed a linear, direct association between phosphate and hemoglobin values, suggesting that the hypophosphatemic impact on hemoglobin (i.e., the reduction in hemoglobin due to hypophosphatemia) could overbear the hyperphosphatemic impact (i.e., the reduction in hemoglobin due to hypophosphatemia).

Several mechanisms could explain our results. First, serum phosphate in dialysis patients is subjected to a quick reduction during the dialysis treatment, due to the low phosphate concentration in the dialysate. Thus, hyperphosphatemia could be adjusted faster than hypophosphatemia, leading to a more stable pathophysiological effect of the latter. Furthermore, the modification in the impact of phosphate on hemoglobin levels in conservative CKD could be due to the increasing FGF23, whose concentration is much higher in hemodialysis (HD) as compared to peritoneal dialysis (PD) or conservative CKD [25]. In addition, in dialysis patients, the association between FGF23 and serum phosphate seems to be less powerful than in patients in conservative treatment [26], and this may be due to the constitutively extremely high level of these hormones in this population, which may lead the body to become accustomed to them. Moreover, the impact of FGF23 on mortality is also reduced in dialysis patients [27]. Finally, serum phosphate augmentation in the interdialytic time represents a chronic process, causing tolerance and compensation mechanisms.

Differently from phosphate, the association between iPTH and anemia has been mainly investigated only in cross-sectional studies [28]. In these studies, PTH has an impact on the hemoglobin level in patients affected by CKD in conservative treatment, but not in dialysis patients. Indeed, in several observational studies in patients affected by CKD in conservative treatment, the PTH seemed to be related to the worse management of anemia, through impairment of the erythrocytes' median of fragility (MOF) and increased EPO resistance [29–31], but few studies were conducted in dialysis patients only. Among these, and in line with our results, no differences in PTH were detected [32].

In keeping with our hypothesis, the association between hemoglobin and age in dialysis also differed from patients in conservative treatment. In detail, whereas hemoglobin is negatively related to age in the majority of studies [33–37], in our cohort, no association was detected. Furthermore, in a univariate longitudinal evaluation, the relationship between hemoglobin and age seemed to be direct, even though not clinically relevant, although in conservatively treated populations, the association is often negative. This highlights the different characteristics of our cohort, which is composed only of dialysis patients, not non-dialysis patients.

Diskin et al. [38] demonstrated that increased ESA doses are needed in patients with hyperphosphatemia. A similar hypothesis was speculated by Kamyar et al. [39] in a cohort of 49,215 patients, showing a significant positive correlation between phosphorus and EPO dose, and confirmed in a multivariate model including "most ESA responsive" and "ESA hyporesponsive" patients. However, as no association between serum phosphate and hemoglobin was tested in this study, this effect could be due to the FGF23 level.

In our analysis, a negative association between ESA and hemoglobin was detected. This could be explained by the fact that, due to the retrospective real-life design of our study, ESA was prescribed only in patients with lower hemoglobin, according to current Clinical Practice Guidelines [40]. For this reason, it can be considered as confounding by indication.

Conversely to the phosphate impact, we found that the assumption of phosphate binder seemed to lightly improve the hemoglobin concentration. This is in line with other studies both in rats [41] and in humans [42,43], which reported an increase in hemoglobin in patients with phosphorous binder. This association, however, could be due to confounding by indication, because phosphate binders are taken by patients with hyperphosphatemia, in turn related to higher hemoglobin. However, even when performing the analysis and excluding phosphate binders from the multivariate model, the results did not differ.

Our study has strengths and limitations. The main strength is the large sample size and the longitudinal design. To our knowledge, no other studies have directly evaluated the association between phosphate and hemoglobin in a large dialysis population. The limitations of our study include the observational design, which cannot exclude the presence of residual confounding, and the absence of information on FGF23 measurements and EPO dose, and also, the iron and ESA type were not detailed in our database. The lack of this information precludes the computation of the ESA hyporesponsiveness index. Furthermore, our analysis included only dialysis patients of Caucasian descent from a single Italian region, thus impairing the generalizability of our study.

5. Conclusions

In conclusion, in our study, performed in a unique large cohort of 6263 dialysis patients, we found that phosphate reduction linearly reduces hemoglobin concentration. This result seems to be independent of personal features, comorbidities, and drugs. In addition, even though our results are not conclusive, age could have an impact on this association. Further studies are needed to confirm this association and to detail if ESA doses can impact on it. Furthermore, the impact of phosphate, hemoglobin, and ESA doses on cardiovascular events and mortality deserve further studies in the future.

Supplementary Materials: The following supporting information can be downloaded at: https://www.mdpi.com/article/10.3390/jcm13195657/s1, Table S1: Baseline correlated of serum phosphate and hemoglobin.; Table S2: Linear Mixed Model showing the direct association between serum phosphate and hemoglobin.; Table S3: Hosmann sensitivity analysis in LMM; Dependent variable: hemoglobin; Figure S1. Diagram for inclusion process.

Author Contributions: Conceptualization, V.C. (Vincenzo Calabrese) and D.S.; methodology, V.C. (Vincenzo Calabrese) and G.L.T.; formal analysis, V.C. (Vincenzo Calabrese), G.L.T. and C.T.; data curation, V.C. (Vincenzo Calabrese), C.T. and V.C. (Valeria Cernaro); writing—original draft preparation, V.C. (Vincenzo Calabrese), C.T. and F.M.-R.; writing—review and editing, V.A.P., S.M., C.T. and V.C. (Valeria Cernaro). All authors have read and agreed to the published version of the manuscript.

Funding: This paper has not received financial support from any institution and represents an original work of the authors.

Institutional Review Board Statement: The study was conducted in accordance with the Declaration of Helsinki and ethical review and approval were waived for this study due the Sicilian Registry of Nephrology, Dialysis, and Transplantation being a collection of regional data, instituted by regional laws. The Sicilian registry was created in 2008, with a decree (03423/08) that established its aim, i.e., collecting data and analyzing it. Informed consent is requested from all patients whose data are entered in the registry. However, as specified in art. 1, no formal approval from ethical committees is needed to analyze data as they are made available only in anonymous form.

Informed Consent Statement: Informed consent was obtained from all subjects involved in the study.

Data Availability Statement: The data were retrieved from the Sicilian Registry of Nephrology, Dialysis, and Transplantation (http://www.crtsicilia.it/PUBLIC/RegistroRSNDT/CentriDialisiETx.aspx (accessed on 6 July 2022)).

Acknowledgments: Data have been kindly provided by the team of the Sicilian Registry of Nephrology, Dialysis and Transplantation.

Conflicts of Interest: The authors declare no conflict of interest. None of the authors has relationships with companies that may have a financial interest in the information contained in the manuscript. I certify that I have answered every question and have not altered the wording of any of the questions on the attached form. This paper has not received financial support from any institution and represents the original work of the authors.

References

1. Rout, P.; Jialal, I. Hyperphosphatemia. In *StatPearls [Internet]*; StatPearls Publishing: Treasure Island, FL, USA, 2024. Available online: https://www.ncbi.nlm.nih.gov/books/NBK551586/ (accessed on 12 June 2023).
2. Cernaro, V.; Santoro, D.; Lucisano, S.; Nicocia, G.; Lacquaniti, A.; Buemi, M. The future of phosphate binders: A perspective on novel therapeutics. *Expert Opin. Investig. Drugs* **2014**, *23*, 1459–1463. [CrossRef] [PubMed]
3. Leifheit-Nestler, M.; Haffner, D. How FGF23 shapes multiple organs in chronic kidney disease. *Mol. Cell. Pediatr.* **2021**, *8*, 12. [CrossRef] [PubMed]
4. Edmonston, D.; Wolf, M. FGF23 at the crossroads of phosphate, iron economy and erythropoiesis. *Nat. Rev. Nephrol.* **2020**, *16*, 7–19. [CrossRef] [PubMed]
5. Fishbane, S.; Spinowitz, B. Update on Anemia in ESRD and Earlier Stages of CKD: Core Curriculum 2018. *Am. J. Kidney Dis. Off. J. Natl. Kidney Found.* **2018**, *71*, 423–435. [CrossRef] [PubMed]
6. Ho, B.B.; Bergwitz, C. FGF23 signalling and physiology. *J. Mol. Endocrinol.* **2021**, *66*, R23–R32. [CrossRef]
7. Ogawa, E.; Kobayashi, K.; Yoshiura, N.; Mukai, J. Bovine postparturient hemoglobinemia: Hypophosphatemia and metabolic disorder in red blood cells. *Am. J. Vet. Res.* **1987**, *48*, 1300–1303.
8. Adams, L.G.; Hardy, R.M.; Weiss, D.J.; Bartges, J.W. Hypophosphatemia and hemolytic anemia associated with diabetes mellitus and hepatic lipidosis in cats. *J. Vet. Intern. Med.* **1993**, *7*, 266–271. [CrossRef]
9. Melvin, J.D.; Watts, R.G. Severe hypophosphatemia: A rare cause of intravascular hemolysis. *Am. J. Hematol.* **2002**, *69*, 223–224. [CrossRef]
10. Jacob, H.S.; Amsden, T. Acute hemolytic anemia with rigid red cells in hypophosphatemia. *N. Engl. J. Med.* **1971**, *285*, 1446–1450. [CrossRef]
11. Young, J.A.; Lichtman, M.A.; Cohen, J. Reduced red cell 2,3-diphosphoglycerate and adenosine triphosphate, hypophosphatemia, and increased hemoglobin-oxygen affinity after cardiac surgery. *Circulation* **1973**, *47*, 1313–1318. [CrossRef]
12. MacDonald, R. Red cell 2,3-diphosphoglycerate and oxygen affinity. *Anaesthesia* **1977**, *32*, 544–553. [CrossRef] [PubMed]
13. Van Kempen TA, T.G.; Deixler, E.; Crook, M.A. Hypophosphatemia as a key factor in sudden infant death syndrome (SIDS)? *Upsala J. Med. Sci.* **2013**, *118*, 143–144. [CrossRef] [PubMed]
14. Shepherd, J.R.; Dominelli, P.B.; Roy, T.K.; Secomb, T.W.; Hoyer, J.D.; Oliveira, J.L.; Joyner, M.J. Modelling the relationships between haemoglobin oxygen affinity and the oxygen cascade in humans. *J. Physiol.* **2019**, *597*, 4193–4202. [CrossRef] [PubMed]
15. Amanzadeh, J.; Reilly, R.F.J. Hypophosphatemia: An evidence-based approach to its clinical consequences and management. *Nat. Clin. Pract. Nephrol.* **2006**, *2*, 136–148. [CrossRef] [PubMed]
16. Farrow, E.G.; Yu, X.; Summers, L.J.; Davis, S.I.; Fleet, J.C.; Allen, M.R.; Robling, A.G.; Stayrook, K.R.; Jideonwo, V.; Magers, M.J.; et al. Iron deficiency drives an autosomal dominant hypophosphatemic rickets (ADHR) phenotype in fibroblast growth factor-23 (Fgf23) knock-in mice. *Proc. Natl. Acad. Sci. USA* **2011**, *108*, E1146–E1155. [CrossRef]
17. Clinkenbeard, E.L.; Farrow, E.G.; Summers, L.J.; Cass, T.A.; Roberts, J.L.; Bayt, C.A.; Lahm, T.; Albrecht, M.; Allen, M.R.; Peacock, M.; et al. Neonatal iron deficiency causes abnormal phosphate metabolism by elevating FGF23 in normal and ADHR mice. *J. Bone Miner. Res.* **2014**, *29*, 361–369. [CrossRef]
18. Kommalapati, A.; Singhi, R.; Tella, S.H. Association between Iron-Deficiency Anemia and Hypophosphatemia. *Am. J. Med.* **2018**, *131*, e103–e104. [CrossRef]
19. Maduell, F.; Navarro, V.; Alós, M.; Torregrosa, E.; Ventura, J.M.; Nicolas, J.; Sanz, M.; Moreno, A. Intradialysis hemolysis secondary to hypophosphatemia. *Nefrologia* **2003**, *23*, 85–88.
20. Lichtman, M.A.; Miller, D.R.; Freeman, R.B. Erythrocyte adenosine triphosphate depletion during hypophosphatemia in a uremic subject. *N. Engl. J. Med.* **1969**, *280*, 240–244. [CrossRef]

21. Centro Regionale Trapianti Sicilia. Available online: http://www.crtsicilia.it/PUBLIC/RegistroRSNDT/CentriDialisiETx.aspx (accessed on 6 July 2022).
22. Czaya, B.; Faul, C. The Role of Fibroblast Growth Factor 23 in Inflammation and Anemia. *Int. J. Mol. Sci.* **2019**, *20*, 4195. [CrossRef] [PubMed]
23. David, V.; Martin, A.; Isakova, T.; Spaulding, C.; Qi, L.; Ramirez, V.; Zumbrennen-Bullough, K.B.; Sun, C.C.; Lin, H.Y.; Babitt, J.L.; et al. Inflammation and functional iron deficiency regulate fibroblast growth factor 23 production. *Kidney Int.* **2016**, *89*, 135–146. [CrossRef] [PubMed]
24. Smith, E.R.; Ford, M.L.; Tomlinson, L.A.; Rajkumar, C.; McMahon, L.P.; Holt, S.G. Phosphorylated fetuin-A-containing calciprotein particles are associated with aortic stiffness and a procalcific milieu in patients with pre-dialysis CKD. *Nephrol. Dial. Transplant.* **2012**, *27*, 1957–1966. [CrossRef]
25. Bi, S.; Liang, Y.; Cheng, L.; Wang, Y.; Wang, T.; Han, Q.; Zhang, A. Hemodialysis is associated with higher serum FGF23 level when compared with peritoneal dialysis. *Int. Urol. Nephrol.* **2017**, *49*, 1653–1659. [CrossRef] [PubMed]
26. Komaba, H.; Fukagawa, M. FGF23: A key player in mineral and bone disorder in CKD. *Nefrologia* **2009**, *29*, 392–396. [PubMed]
27. Olauson, H.; Qureshi, A.R.; Miyamoto, T.; Barany, P.; Heimburger, O.; Lindholm, B.; Stenvinkel, P.; Larsson, T.E. Relation between serum fibroblast growth factor-23 level and mortality in incident dialysis patients: Are gender and cardiovascular disease confounding the relationship? *Nephrol. Dial. Transplant.* **2010**, *25*, 3033–3038. [CrossRef]
28. Tran, L.; Batech, M.; Rhee, C.M.; Streja, E.; Kalantar-Zadeh, K.; Jacobsen, S.J.; Sim, J.J. Serum phosphorus and association with anemia among a large diverse population with and without chronic kidney disease. *Nephrol. Dial. Transplant.* **2016**, *31*, 636–645. [CrossRef]
29. Bogin, E.; Massry, S.G.; Levi, J.; Djaldeti, M.; Bristol, G.; Smith, J. Effect of parathyroid hormone on osmotic fragility of human erythrocytes. *J. Clin. Investig.* **1982**, *69*, 1017–1025. [CrossRef]
30. Ureña, P.; Eckardt, K.U.; Sarfati, E.; Zingraff, J.; Zins, B.; Roullet, J.B.; Roland, E.; Drüeke, T.; Kurtz, A. Serum erythropoietin and erythropoiesis in primary and secondary hyperparathyroidism: Effect of parathyroidectomy. *Nephron* **1991**, *59*, 384–393. [CrossRef]
31. Zingraff, J.; Drüeke, T.; Marie, P.; Man, N.K.; Jungers, P.; Bordier, P. Anemia and secondary hyperparathyroidism. *Arch. Intern. Med.* **1978**, *138*, 1650–1652. [CrossRef]
32. Bal, Z.; Demirci, B.G.; Karakose, S.; Tutal, E.; Erkmen Uyar, M.; Acar, N.O.; Sezer, S. Factors Influencing Hemoglobin Variability and Its Association with Mortality in Hemodialysis Patients. *Sci. World J.* **2018**, *2018*, 8065691. [CrossRef] [PubMed]
33. García-Erce, J.A.; Lorente-Aznar, T.; Rivilla-Marugán, L. Influence of gender, age and residence altitude on haemoglobin levels and the prevalence of anaemia. *Med. Clin.* **2019**, *153*, 424–429. [CrossRef] [PubMed]
34. Gómez Ramírez, S.; Remacha Sevilla, Á.F.; Muñoz Gómez, M. Anaemia in the elderly. *Med. Clin.* **2017**, *149*, 496–503. [CrossRef] [PubMed]
35. Blum, L.V.; Schmitt, E.; Choorapoikayil, S.; Baumhove, O.; Bayer, A.; Friederich, P.; Friedrich, J.; Geisen, C.; Gruenewald, M.; Gutjahr, M.; et al. Association of anaemia, co-morbidities and red blood cell transfusion according to age groups: Multicentre sub-analysis of the German Patient Blood Management Network Registry. *BJS Open* **2022**, *6*, zrac128. [CrossRef]
36. Robalo Nunes, A.; Fonseca, C.; Marques, F.; Belo, A.; Brilhante, D.; Cortez, J. Prevalence of anemia and iron deficiency in older Portuguese adults: An EMPIRE substudy. *Geriatr. Gerontol. Int.* **2017**, *17*, 1814–1822. [CrossRef]
37. Guralnik, J.M.; Eisenstaedt, R.S.; Ferrucci, L.; Klein, H.G.; Woodman, R.C. Prevalence of anemia in persons 65 years and older in the United States: Evidence for a high rate of unexplained anemia. *Blood* **2004**, *104*, 2263–2268. [CrossRef]
38. Diskin, C.J.; Stokes, T.J.; Dansby, L.M.; Radcliff, L.; Carter, T.B. Can acidosis and hyperphosphataemia result in increased erythropoietin dosing in haemodialysis patients? *Nephrology* **2006**, *11*, 394–399. [CrossRef]
39. Kalantar-Zadeh, K.; Lee, G.H.; Miller, J.E.; Streja, E.; Jing, J.; Robertson, J.A.; Kovesdy, C.P. Predictors of hyporesponsiveness to erythropoiesis-stimulating agents in hemodialysis patients. *Am. J. Kidney Dis.* **2009**, *53*, 823–834. [CrossRef]
40. McMurray, J.; Parfrey, P.; Adamson, J.W.; Aljama, P.; Berns, J.S.; Bohlius, J.; Drüeke, T.B.; Finkelstein, F.O.; Fishbane, S.; Ganz, T.; et al. Kidney Disease: Improving Global Outcomes (KDIGO) Anemia Work Group—KDIGO Clinical Practice Guideline for Anemia in Chronic Kidney Disease. *Kidney Int. Suppl.* **2012**, *2*, 279–335.
41. Vaziri, N.D.; Nunes, A.C.; Said, H.; Khazaeli, M.; Liu, H.; Zhao, Y.; Jing, W.; Cogburn, K.; Alikhani, L.; Lau, W.L. Route of intestinal absorption and tissue distribution of iron contained in the novel phosphate binder ferric citrate. *Nephrol. Dial. Transplant.* **2020**, *35*, 1136–1144. [CrossRef]
42. Maruyama, N.; Otsuki, T.; Yoshida, Y.; Nagura, C.; Kitai, M.; Shibahara, N.; Tomita, H.; Maruyama, T.; Abe, M. Ferric Citrate Decreases Fibroblast Growth Factor 23 and Improves Erythropoietin Responsiveness in Hemodialysis Patients. *Am. J. Nephrol.* **2018**, *47*, 406–414. [CrossRef] [PubMed]
43. Shima, H.; Miya, K.; Okada, K.; Minakuchi, J.; Kawashima, S. Sucroferric oxyhydroxide decreases serum phosphorus level and fibroblast growth factor 23 and improves renal anemia in hemodialysis patients. *BMC Res. Notes* **2018**, *11*, 363. [CrossRef] [PubMed]

Journal of
Clinical Medicine

MDPI

Article

Rationale and Protocol of the ETERNITY-ITA Study: Use of Etelcalcetide for Preserving Vitamin K-Dependent Protein Activity—An Italian Study

Maria Fusaro [1,2,*], Andrea Aghi [3], Carmela Marino [4], Francesca Mallamaci [4,5], Mario Plebani [6], Martina Zaninotto [6], Maria Grano [7], Silvia Colucci [8], Maurizio Gallieni [9,10,11], Thomas L. Nickolas [12], Sandro Giannini [13], Stefania Sella [13], Paolo Simioni [13], Alberto Bazzocchi [14], Giuseppe Guglielmi [15], Fulvia Taddei [16], Enrico Schileo [16], Maria Carmela Versace [4] and Giovanni Tripepi [4,†] for the ETERNITY-ITA Study Investigators

1 National Research Council (CNR), Institute of Clinical Physiology (IFC), 56124 Pisa, Italy
2 Department of Medicine, University of Padova, 35128 Padova, Italy
3 Independent Researcher, 35128 Padua, Italy; andrea.aghi@gmail.com
4 Research Unit of Clinical Epidemiology of Reggio Calabria, Institute of Clinical Physiology (IFC), National Research Council (CNR), 89124 Reggio Calabria, Italy; cmarino@ifc.cnr.it (C.M.); francesca.mallamaci@libero.it (F.M.); mcversace@ifc.cnr.it (M.C.V.)
5 Nephrology, Dialysis and Transplantation Unit, Grande Ospedale Metropolitano, Bianchi-Melacrino-Morelli (BMM), 89124 Reggio Calabria, Italy
6 QI.LAB.MED, Spin-Off of the University of Padova, 35011 Campodarsego, Italy; mario.plebani@unipd.it (M.P.); martina.zaninotto@aopd.veneto.it (M.Z.)
7 Department of Precision and Regenerative Medicine and Ionian Area, University of Bari, Piazza Giulio Cesare 11, 70124 Bari, Italy; maria.grano@uniba.it
8 Department of Translational Biomedicine and Neuroscience, University of Bari, 70124 Bari, Italy; silviaconcetta.colucci@uniba.it
9 Department of Biomedical and Clinical Sciences 'Luigi Sacco', Università di Milano, 20157 Milano, Italy; maurizio.gallieni@unimi.it
10 Post-Graduate School of Specialization in Nephrology, University of Milano, 20157 Milano, Italy
11 Division of Nephrology and Dialysis, Azienda Socio-Sanitaria Territoriale (ASST) Fatebenefratelli-Sacco, Fatebenefratelli Hospital, 20157 Milan, Italy
12 Department of Medicine, Division of Nephrology, Columbia University, New York, NY 10032, USA; tln2001@cumc.columbia.edu
13 Department of Medicine, Clinica Medica 1, University of Padova, 35128 Padova, Italy; sandro.giannini@unipd.it (S.G.); stefania.sella@unipd.it (S.S.); paolo.simioni@unipd.it (P.S.)
14 Diagnostic and Interventional Radiology, IRCCS Istituto Ortopedico Rizzoli, 40136 Bologna, Italy; abazzocchi@gmail.com
15 Department of Clinical and Experimental Medicine, Foggia University School of Medicine, 71122 Foggia, Italy; giuseppe.guglielmi@unifg.it
16 Bioengineering and Computing Laboratory, IRCCS Istituto Ortopedico Rizzoli, 40136 Bologna, Italy; fulvia.taddei@ior.it (F.T.); enrico.schileo@ior.it (E.S.)
* Correspondence: dante.lucia11@gmail.com
† Investigators of the ETERNITY-ITA is provided in the Acknowledgments.

Abstract: Background/Objectives: Chronic kidney disease and mineral bone disorders (CKD-MBD) are frequently associated with an increased risk of both vascular calcifications (VCs) and bone fractures (BFs). The complex pathogenesis of VCs and BFs involves various factors such as calcium overload, phosphate imbalance, and secondary hyperparathyroidism. Key players, such as the vitamin K-dependent proteins (VKDPs) matrix Gla protein (MGP) and bone Gla protein (BGP), have pivotal roles both for VCs and BFs. The VIKI study highlighted that hemodialysis patients treated with calcimimetics had higher levels of total BGP and MGP compared to those untreated, suggesting a potential protective effect of these drugs on BFs and VCs beyond the beneficial effect of reducing PTH levels. **Methods:** ETERNITY-ITA is a multi-center, comparative effectiveness, observational, longitudinal study that will enroll 160 hemodialysis patients (80 patients treated with Etelcalcetide and 80 age- and sex-matched patients treated with calcitriol or vitamin D analogs). Nephrologists will tailor the target dose of Etelcalcetide on an individual level to achieve the KDIGO PTH target. In the Etelcalcetide-treated group, the addition of calcitriol will be allowed when required by clinical practice (for correction of hypocalcemia). **Conclusions:** This study will evaluate the real-world effect of Etelcalcetide on VKDP levels, such as BGP and MGP, at 3, 9, and 18 months from baseline. The resulting preservation of vascular and bone health will be assessed for the first time by examining aortic and iliac artery calcifications and vertebral fractures, respectively.

Keywords: bone fractures; etecalcetide; hemodialysis; vascular calcification; vitamin K

1. Introduction

Vascular calcifications (VCs) are common complication of CKD mineral and bone disorders (CKD-MBD). In CKD patients, the prevalence of aortic calcification is higher than in the general population and VCs were found to be associated with a higher prevalence of bone fractures (BFs) [1]. The pathogenesis of VC in CKD patients is multifactorial, with calcium and phosphate overload and secondary hyperparathyroidism (HPT) among the most relevant etiological factors [2]. Calcification inhibitors are also important determinants of VCs [3]. A vitamin K-dependent protein (VKDP), such as matrix Gla protein (MGP), is characterized not only by five sites of carboxylation (c-MGP) but also by the phosphorylation of three serine residues (p-c MGP, through the enzyme casein kinase) [4,5], which seem to regulate protein secretion into the extracellular environment [5]. The main function of MGP is associated with the carboxylate form, which makes it a strong inhibitor of vascular calcifications, probably due to its interaction with bone morphogenetic protein 2 (BMP-2: a powerful osteoinductive protein), which transforms vascular smooth muscle cells (VSMCs) into osteoblast-like cells [6]. c-MGP binds calcification crystals in blood vessels, forming vesicles and apoptotic bodies and preventing both calcium phosphate precipitation and the trans-differentiation of VSMCs into an osteogenic phenotype [5]. Another remarkable VKDP is bone Gla protein (BGP), which is mainly secreted by osteoblasts and in small quantities even by chondrocytes [7,8]. It has three carboxylated sites, making it active in its main bone mineralization action and allowing the interaction between the calcium-binding Gla residues and the calcium ions of hydroxyapatite, forming hydroxyapatite crystals. Indeed, BGP also acts as an inhibitor of bone mineralization, regulating mineral maturation [8].

The current paradigm for reducing the risk of vascular calcification (VC) development and progression revolves around the reduction of parathyroid hormone (PTH), calcium, and phosphorus. In particular, the recent Kidney Disease Improving Global Outcomes (KDIGO) guidelines recommend targeting PTH levels to a range between 2–9 times the upper normal limit [2]. In this scenario, Etelcalcetide emerges as a novel synthetic peptide that binds the calcium-sensing receptor-enhancing activation of the receptor itself through extracellular calcium and at the same time decreases PTH secretion in parathyroid cells [9]. Experimental studies [1] and human studies [7] have shown that oral calcimimetics use prevents vascular calcification by an MGP-mediated mechanism (increasing MGP serum levels) not seen with the use of vitamin D or its analogs.

The main aim of this study will be to assess whether Etelcalcetide, compared to vitamin D or vitamin D analog treatments, increases the levels of vitamin K-dependent proteins (VKDPs) such as bone Gla protein (BGP) and matrix Gla protein (MGP) at 3, 9, and 18 months from baseline, resulting in proper bone mineralization and inhibition of vascular calcification. The secondary aims include evaluating, at 18 months, whether treatment with Etelcalcetide decreases the progression of vascular calcification (in the aorta and iliac arteries) and vertebral fractures.

2. Methods

2.1. Study Design

This is a national, multi-center, comparative effectiveness, observational, longitudinal study with no predefined interference on drug dosing by the investigators. Nineteen Italian centers will be involved. In each center, 14 patients will be screened for eligibility and about 10–12 patients are scheduled to be enrolled. This study will enroll 160 hemodialysis patients (80 patients treated with Etelcalcetide and 80 age- and sex-matched patients treated with calcitriol or a vitamin D analog, paricalcitol) (Figure 1).

Participants	Treatment
Exposed group, n=80 Every study participant who complies with inclusion/exclusion criteria and receives Etelcalcetide prescribed by their treating physician according to current clinical practice will be included in the exposed group.	**Drug: Etelcalcetide** Administered intravenously at the end of each dialysis session. Dosing ranges from 2.5 mg to 15 mg set by the patient's physician. **Other Name: Parsabiv**
Unexposed group, n=80 Every study participant who complies with the inclusion/exclusion criteria and receives oral calcitriol or vitamin D analogs (paricalcitol) prescribed by their treating physician according to current clinical practice will be included in the unexposed group. Patients of this group will be matched (1:1) to patients of the exposed group as for age and gender.	**Drug:** **Vitamin D or Vitamin D analogs (paricalcitol)**

Figure 1. Study groups.

Given the observational nature of this study, the investigators will not recommend target goals of Etelcalcetide treatment. The treating nephrologists will tailor their target dose of Etelcalcetide on an individual-level patient basis in order to achieve the KDIGO PTH target levels. In the Etelcalcetide-treated group, the addition of calcitriol is allowed when required by current clinical practice (for correction of hypocalcemia). Blood samples for the measurement of specific biomarkers will be collected in concomitance with the routine blood sampling scheduled in each center. At baseline, all relevant demographic, clinical, and biochemical data will be collected in compliance with the privacy laws of the European Union. The study design is illustrated in Figure 2.

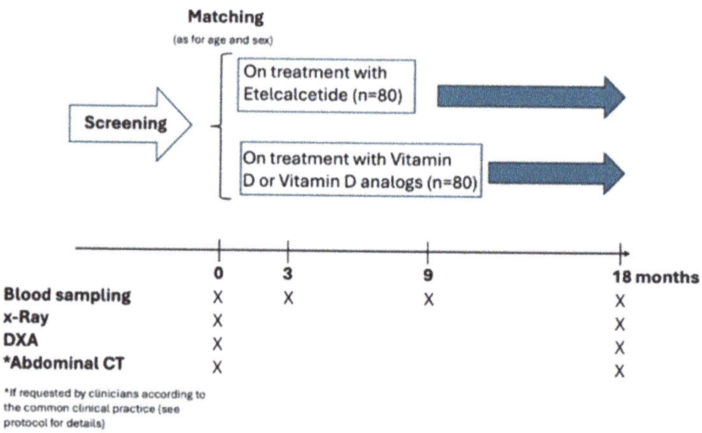

Figure 2. Graphical representation of the study protocol.

2.2. Ethical Considerations

Written informed consent will be obtained from each participant. The study is registered at clinicaltrials.gov: NCT 06352957. This study will be conducted according to the Helsinki declaration.

3. Study Objectives and Aims

3.1. Main Outcome Measures

The main outcome measure is the comparison of VKDP levels between patients treated with Etelcalcetide and those treated with vitamin D or vitamin D analogs. The longitudinal changes of the following VKDPs (measured at baseline and after 3, 9, and 18 months) will be compared between the two groups: total MGP, dephosphorylated-undercarboxylated MGP (dp-ucMGP), total BGP, and undercarboxylated BGP (ucBGP).

3.2. Other Outcome Measures

1. The following bone vascular marker levels will be considered: calcium, phosphate, magnesium, ALP, PTH, 25(OH)D, procollagen I intact N-terminal or P1NP, C-terminal telopeptide or CTX, tartrate-resistant acid phosphatase 5b or TRAP 5bC-Terminal to Intact, bone-specific alkaline phosphatase (BSAP), fibroblast growth factor 23 or cFGF23 and iFGF23, klotho and soluble α-klotho, sclerostin and bioactive sclerostin, DKK1, fetuin-A, zinc, and irisin.

   The analysis will assess whether Etelcalcetide will affect the levels of the above-mentioned biomarkers over time.

2. Evaluation of serum calcification propensity using the T50 test [10,11].
3. Changes from baseline of the following anemia marker levels are considered: hemoglobin (Hb), hematocrit (Ht), plates (PLTS), reticulocytes, iron, ferritin, transferrin, and transferrin saturation. This is to test whether 3, 9, and 18 months of treatment with Etelcalcetide improves anemia status (e.g., reduced EPO and/or iron doses).
4. Changes from baseline of the following dialysis routine biomarkers: albumin, KT/V, aluminum, C-reactive protein (CRP), cholesterol, triglycerides, cholesterol HDL, and cholesterol LDL.

   The analysis will assess whether Etelcalcetide will affect the levels of the above-mentioned biomarkers over time.

5. Changes from baseline prevalence VCs (aorta and iliac arteries) measured using a lateral dorsal lumbar spine X-ray [time frame: 18 months].

   To test whether 18 months of treatment with Etelcalcetide reduces VC progression.

6. Changes from the baseline prevalence of vertebral fractures (VFs, quantitative vertebral morphometry using dedicated software, Optasia Medical SpineAnalyzer 4.0, version 4.0.2.19) measured using a lateral dorsal lumbar spine X-ray [time frame: 18 months].

   To test whether 18 months of treatment with Etelcalcetide reduces VF progression.

7. Changes from baseline total hip, femoral, and neck bone mass density (BMD), measured by dual-energy X-ray absorptiometry (DEXA), including a trabecular bone score (TBS) when available. To test if 18 months of treatment with Etelcalcetide improves BMD and TBS.
8. To assess the relationship of bone vascular biomarkers and clinical outcomes: VFs and VCs.
9. To compare a novel quantitative computer-assisted scoring method for vascular calcifications with a three-dimensional assessment from CT data [12,13].
10. To evaluate the effect of Etelcalcetide on cardiovascular events and all-cause mortality.
11. To evaluate the safety of Etelcalcetide and drug interactions.

3.3. Inclusion Criteria

1. Patient has provided informed consent.
2. Patient is 18 years of age or older of both sexes.
3. Patients receiving maintenance HD three times per week (Kt/V >1.2).
4. Parathyroid hormone concentrations >500 ng/l at screening, or if parathyroidectomy is planned or expected, Ca >8.3 mg/dL.
5. Will be considered in the exposed group:
    a. patients who have started Etelcalcetide within 1 month of study enrolment;
    b. patients naïve to intravenous calcimimetics use;
    c. patients who have suspended oral calcimimetics for at least 1 month;
    d. patients who are not responding to or non-compliant with treatment with calcitriol.
6. In the unexposed group, patients being treated with calcitriol or vitamin D analogs and who are age- (±2 years) and sex-comparable (matching) to those in the exposed group will be considered.
7. Native vitamin D can be used in both groups and should be administered to target a 25(OH)D level >30 ng/mL.
8. Dialysate calcium concentration must be stable for at least 4 weeks prior to screening laboratory assessments.
9. Patient must have severe HPT as defined by two laboratory screening pre-dialysis serum PTH values >500 pg/mL, measured on two consecutive lab checks prior to entering the study. PTH levels should be standardized as reported elsewhere [14].
10. Total alkaline phosphatase greater than the normal range, or even within the normal range but if greater than the tertile of the reference range for the assay.
11. Patients will be eligible only if they will show at least moderate aorta VCs [15] and/or iliac artery VCs and at least a mild VF [16,17].

3.4. Exclusion Criteria

1. Previous treatment with oral calcimimetics (cinacalcet) must have been suspended for at least 30 days. Recent start of calcimimetics (Etelcalcetide) is acceptable, but patients are excluded if the treatment lasts for more than 1 month.
2. Patients who received a bisphosphonate, denosumab, or teriparatide during the 12 months prior to screening.
3. Patients who underwent parathyroidectomy in the 6 months before the start of the study or if the procedure is scheduled soon.
4. Scheduled kidney transplant during the study period or anticipated living donor evaluation within three months of recruitment.
5. Patients with unstable medical conditions based on medical history, physical examinations, and routine laboratory tests, or otherwise deemed unstable in the judgment of the Investigator.
6. Having metabolic bone diseases not related to the kidney (i.e., Pagets, Osteogenesis Imperfecta).
7. With severe untreated hyperthyroidism.
8. With malignancy within the last 3 years (except non-melanoma skin cancers or cervical carcinoma in situ).
9. Patients pregnant or nursing.
10. Patients with Long QT Syndrome.
11. Patients who are unlikely to be available to complete all protocol-required study visits or procedures, and/or to comply with all required study procedures to the best of the patient's and Investigator's knowledge.

4. Statistical Considerations

4.1. Sample Size

One hundred and sixty patients on hemodialysis are needed to address the study hypothesis. The sample size was established on pragmatic grounds by considering the statistical models that will be applied to address the study hypothesis [i.e., the linear mixed models (LMM) analysis or generalized estimating equations (GEE)]. In this case, a total of 640 observations over the time period will be collected in 160 patients, thus ensuring adequate power to adjust for major potential confounders.

4.2. Data Analysis

Normally distributed variables will be summarized as means and standard deviations, non-normally distributed variables as medians and interquartile ranges, and categorical data as absolute numbers and percentages. At baseline, the between-groups comparisons will be performed using the independent *t*-Test, the Mann–Whitney U Test, or the Chi-squared test, as appropriate. The between-groups comparisons of repeated measurements of biomarkers (as continuous variables) over time will be performed by linear mixed models (LMM) or generalized estimating equations (GEE). No imputation method of missing values will be applied. In these analyses, the effect of the exposure to Etelcalcetide in treated patients versus those untreated will be preliminarily investigated by including the group variable, the time, and the interaction term between the group variable and time. The effect of potential confounders on the effectiveness of Etelcalcetide on the study outcomes will be further investigated by adjusting for all potential confounders, including medications, by multiple regression models. Sensitivity analysis by applying the propensity score approach will be also performed. The primary analysis will be conducted considering the patients as belonging to the treatment arm they had at the beginning of observation. A secondary analysis will also be performed taking into account any cross-over. Survival analyses will be performed using the Kaplan–Meier and Cox regression methods. All statistical analyses will be performed using a standard statistical package (STATA 16, StataCorp. Stata Statistical Software. College Station, TX, USA).

5. Laboratories and Instrumental Data

The following laboratory testing will be performed:

- As part of current clinical practice, the following routine biomarkers, such as calcium, phosphate, magnesium, ALP, PTH, 25(OH)D, Hb, Ht, PLTS, reticulocytes, Fe, ferritin, transferrin, and transferrin saturation, will be measured in each participating center.
- Specific bone vascular markers (which will be measured in a centralized laboratory) considered are total MGP and BGP, dp-ucMGP, ucBGP, procollagen I intact N-terminal or P1NP, C-terminal telopeptide or CTX, tartrate-resistant acid phosphatase 5b or TRAP 5bC-Terminal to Intact, bone-specific alkaline phosphatase (BSAP), fibroblast growth factor 23 or cFGF23 and iFGF23, klotho and soluble α-klotho, sclerostin and bioactive sclerostin, DKK1, fetuin-A, and Zinc.

5.1. Instrumental Data

5.1.1. X-ray

According to the current indications of good clinical practice and guidelines, at baseline, the patients will undergo a lateral dorsal lumbar spine X-ray using dedicated software (Calcify 2D [13]) to evaluate vascular calcifications (VCs: aorta and iliac arteries) [12–15] and VFs, where vertebral fractures will be identified if the height of the vertebral body is reduced by at least 20% or 4 mm, according to Genant et al. [16]. Furthermore, a lateral dorsal lumbar spine X-ray will be performed at the end of follow-up at 18 months. Both VCs and VFs will be assessed independently by two physicians who are blinded to the patient's clinical characteristics.

5.1.2. DXA

According to the current indications of good clinical practice and guidelines [2], at baseline, measurements of total hip, femoral, and neck bone mineral density (BMD) will be assessed by dual-energy X-ray absorptiometry (DXA), including a trabecular bone score

(TBS) when available. Furthermore, DXA and TBS will be performed at the end of follow-up at 18 months.

5.1.3. Abdominal CT

If the physician, in the case of the presence of moderate/severe aorta VCs associated with co-morbidity with a resulting higher risk of cardiovascular and mortality events, prescribes an abdominal CT, these findings will be included in the study as data reflecting common clinical practice. In addition, a subset of patients with aorta calcifications confirmed by X-rays will undergo CT scans of the lumbar spine. According to [12], calcification will be considered to be present if an area of $\geq$1 mm^2 displays a density of $\geq$130 Hounsfield units. The AAC score will be calculated from the takeoff of the renal artery to the bifurcation of the aorta into the common iliac arteries. The cross-section of the abdominal aorta on each slice will be divided radially into 12 segments. The abdominal aortic calcification index (ACI) will be calculated as follows: ACI = (total score for calcification in all slices)/ 12 $\times$ 1/(number of slices) $\times$ 100 (%). Semi-quantitative measurement of AAC on lateral X-rays will be conducted independently by two physicians who are blinded to the patient's clinical characteristics. The general description of this study (including the types of clinical examinations and blood sampling over time) is given in Figure 2.

6. Preliminary Results

In a previous paper by us [7], we measured BGP and MGP levels and checked for the presence of vertebral fractures and vascular calcifications using a lateral dorsal lumbar spine X-ray through dedicated software (Optasia Medical SpineAnalyzer 4.0, version 4.0.2.19) to evaluate VFs, which were identified by a height vertebral reduction of at least 20% or 4 mm, according to Genant et al. [16]. In the same X-ray, we evaluated vascular calcifications (VCs: aorta and iliac arteries) [7] in 387 hemodialysis patients enrolled in the VIKI study. Total BGP levels were found to be twice as high in patients on calcimimetics compared to those untreated with this drug class (290 vs. 158.5 mcg/L, $p < 0.0001$), whereas total MGP levels were 19% higher in patients on calcimimetics (21.5 vs. 18.1 mcg/L, $p = 0.04$) than in the untreated group. Median total BGP levels were 29% lower in patients with one or more vertebral fractures (151 vs. 213 mcg/L, $p = 0.0091$) and 36% lower in patients with vascular calcifications (164 vs. 262.1 mcg/L, $p = 0.0003$). In non-survivors, median BGP and MGP levels were lower, but only the difference in MGP levels reached statistical significance (152 vs. 191 mcg/L, $p = 0.20$ and 15.0 vs. 19.7 mcg/L, $p = 0.02$, respectively). In another paper by our group [18], we assessed the prevalence of vitamin K deficiency and the relationship between vitamin K status, vertebral fractures, and vascular calcification in the same patient cohort. Overall, we found a relatively high proportion of patients with deficiencies in MK7 (35.4%), vitamin K1 (23.5%), and MK4 (14.5%). Of note, vitamin K1 deficiency was the strongest predictor of vertebral fractures (odds ratio [OR], 2.94; 95% confidence interval [CI], 1.38–6.26). MK4 deficiency was a predictor of aortic calcification (OR, 2.82; 95% CI, 1.14–7.01), whereas MK5 deficiency appeared to protect against it (OR, 0.38; 95% CI, 0.15–0.95). MK7 deficiency was a predictor of iliac calcification (OR, 1.64; 95% CI, 1.03–2.60). The presence of vertebral fractures was also a predictor of vascular calcifications (OR, 1.76; 95% CI, 1.00–3.08).

7. Discussion

In addition to its known suppressive effect on PTH, Etelcalcetide has demonstrated additional benefits in recent studies, both experimental and human. In rats, it has been shown to preserve cortical bone structure and bone strength by lowering PTH in subtotal Nx rats with established SHPT [19,20]. In humans, it has been found to improve areal bone mineral density and trabecular quality in the central skeleton, always by lowering bone turnover without affecting bone material properties, thereby reducing the risk of fractures [21,22]. A recent meta-analysis comparing various calcimimetics has shown that Etelcalcetide is the most efficacious calcimimetic agent for lowering serum PTH levels but highlighted side effects such as hypocalcemia, nausea, and vomiting. Cinacalcet ranked worst for nausea and had somewhat lower effectiveness, while Evocalcet (in use in Asian populations) had lower effectiveness for decreasing PTH levels but was associated with fewer adverse effects [23].

Ca^{2+}-sensing receptors (CaSRs) are broadly expressed in the vascular system, including perivascular neurons, vascular endothelial cells (VECs), and vascular smooth muscle cells (VSMCs). Prolonged serum calcium is thought to reduce the sensitivity and expression of CaSR in arteries, thereby increasing intra-vascular Ca^{2+} concentrations through a negative feedback loop. Excess intravascular calcium gradually deposits in VSMCs and may in part lead to the transformation of VSMCs into osteoblast-like cells, leading to the formation of vascular calcification [24]. In experimental studies, overexpression of the CaSR reduced the deposition of calcium in human aortic smooth muscle cells (HASMCs) [24]. In uremic rats with secondary HPT treated with calcimimetics (R-568 or AMG 641), compared to the untreated mice, Rodriguez et al. reported that VCs were prevented and mortality was reduced in excess of what was expected from a reduction in calcium and phosphorus alone [25]. They have also ascribed a protective role to calcimimetics as they play a role in the expression of proteins that prevent the development of VCs, in particular highlighting an increase in MGP and a resulting reduction in osteoblastic gene expression markers such as BMP2 [7,25,26]. To confirm these findings, our group conducted a secondary analysis of the Vitamin K Italian (VIKI) study to assess the prevalence of vitamin K deficiency in hemodialysis patients [18] and to evaluate associations between drug consumption and VKDP levels in 387 hemodialyzed patients [7]. A previous study by us reported, in patients managed with calcimimetics compared to without calcimimetics, that total BGP levels were twice as high (290 vs. 158.5 mcg/L, $p < 0.0001$) and that total MGP levels were 19% higher (21.5 vs. 18.1 mcg/L, $p = 0.04$) [7,18]. Furthermore, Yu et al. showed lower aorta calcium content in uremic rats treated with Etelcalcetide than in paricalcitol-treated rats [27]. The precise mechanism by which calcimimetics enhance VKDP activity remains unclear.

Furthermore, recent studies have also shown that irisin, the hormone-like myokine crucial for muscle-bone communication [28], was significantly lower in hemodialysis patients compared with control subjects. Most importantly, within the group of hemodialysis patients, irisin was significantly lower in those with VCs compared to patients with no calcification [29].

7.1. Statistical and Methodological Issues

The study protocol rests on a solid longitudinal design, contemplating repeated measurements of specific biomarkers over time. When dealing with an observational study of effectiveness and with LMM/GEE (see Statistical Analysis) having repeated measurements over time as dependent variables, the estimation of the sample size mainly depends on the number of potential confounders to be included in the models rather than on a predefined effect of the drug. In this case, a total of 640 observations over the time period are expected to be collected [i.e., 80 patients x four longitudinal visits including baseline (n = 320 observations) in the exposed group and 80 patients x four longitudinal visits including baseline (n = 320 observations) in the unexposed group]. This high number of observations will allow us to adjust the effect of Etelcalcetide versus calcitriol or vitamin D analogs on study endpoints for both baseline and longitudinal potential confounders, thus obtaining robust and precise effect estimates. Furthermore, linear mixed models and generalized estimating equations analyses are robust methods for dealing with various patterns of missingness, an issue of particular relevance in studies of comparative effectiveness. Furthermore, since this is not an interventional study, the observational nature of the protocol will be guaranteed by inviting treating nephrologists to tailor the appropriate dosage for each patient individually, aiming to reach the KDIGO PTH target level as in everyday clinical practice. In the group receiving Etelcalcetide, calcitriol may also be added as needed according to the standard clinical approach to address hypocalcemia.

7.2. Dissemination Plan

The target audience to disseminate the results of the ETERNITY-ITA study includes healthcare professionals (nephrologists, endocrinologists, and general practitioners), patients suffering from chronic kidney disease and related conditions, pharmaceutical companies involved in the production of Etelcalcetide and calcitriol, and policy-makers and regulatory bodies involved in healthcare decision-making. The dissemination channels include scientific journals, national and international meetings, and online platforms such as ResearchGate, LinkedIn, and professional forums.

7.3. Limitations

As an observational study of comparative effectiveness, ETERNITY-ITA can provide valuable insights into how treatments perform in real-world settings. However, the observational design comes with limitations that can affect the reliability and validity of the findings, such as those due to confounding. However, such problems will be minimized by collecting data and adjusting for major potential confounders that may interfere with the pathway between treatments and outcome variables. Notwithstanding such an approach aimed at controlling for confounding variables, it is not possible to completely exclude that there may be unmeasured confounders that remain unaccounted for, leading to residual confounding and potentially biased estimates of treatment effects.

8. Conclusions

The clinical remarkable significance of this study is to provide first-time data on the ability of Etelcalcetide in real life to prevent increased VKDP levels, alone or in association with other vascular bone markers, such as skeletal fragility and vascular calcifications, in hemodialysis patients, with a resulting decrease in morbidity and mortality.

Author Contributions: Conceptualization: M.F. and G.T.; Data curation: A.A. and M.C.V.; Formal analysis: M.F., G.T., A.A., F.T. and E.S.; Investigation: G.T., A.B. and G.G.; Methodology: A.A., G.T. and M.G. (Maurizio Gallieni); Project administration: M.F.; Resources: M.P., M.Z., M.G. (Maria Grano) and S.C.; Software: F.T., E.S., M.C.V., A.B. and G.G.; Supervision: M.F., M.Z., M.P., C.M., S.C., M.G. (Maria Grano), M.G. (Maurizio Gallieni), T.L.N., S.G., S.S. and P.S.; Validation: M.F., F.M., T.L.N., S.G., S.S. and P.S.; Writing—original draft: M.F. and G.T.; Writing—review & editing: M.P., M.Z., F.M., A.A., F.T., E.S., C.M., S.C., M.G. (Maria Grano), M.G. (Maurizio Gallieni), T.L.N., S.G., S.S., P.S, A.B. and G.G. All authors have read and agreed to the published version of the manuscript.

Funding: This research received no external funding.

Institutional Review Board Statement: The authors are committed to obtaining informed consent from all participants involved in ETERNITY-ITA. Prior to their participation, participants will be provided with clear and comprehensible information regarding the nature of the study, its objectives, potential risks and benefits, and their rights as participants. The authors will ensure that participants have the opportunity to ask questions and make informed decisions about their participation, without any form of coercion or undue influence. The data collection will strictly adhere to protocols for data anonymization and encryption to safeguard the identity of participants. All data collected by RED-CAP will be securely stored and accessible only to authorized members of the research team. Any identifiable information will be removed or coded to prevent identification of individual participants. Any potential risks will be disclosed to participants during the informed consent process, and steps will be taken to minimize these risks to the greatest extent possible. The study complies with all relevant regulations, guidelines, and ethical standards governing research involving human participants. The authors will obtain necessary approvals from institutional review boards or ethics committees prior to the commencement of the study and will adhere to all applicable laws and regulations regarding the collection, use, and dissemination of data, and obtain necessary permissions for any secondary use of data. Written informed consent will be obtained for each subject. The trial is registered at clinicaltrials.gov: NCT 06352957. The study will be conducted in accordance with the Declaration of Helsinki, and was approved by the Institutional Review Board (or Ethics Committee) of Grande Ospedale Metropolitano BMM of Reggio Calabria, Italy (protocol code RC23022022—23/02/20221)" for studies involving humans.

Informed Consent Statement: Informed consent was obtained from all subjects involved in the study.

Data Availability Statement: Data are contained within the article.

Acknowledgments: The authors thank the ETERNITY-ITA Study Investigators, who will provide patient clinical care and collect clinical data. They are the following: Abaterusso Cataldo, Favaro Enrico (Castelfranco Veneto), Bosco Manuela, Barbecar Dorina (Gorizia-Monfalcone), Dattolo Pietro, Tsalouchos Aris (Firenze), Dugo Mauro, Gresa Baboci (Mestre, Venezia), Gallieni Maurizio, Cosmai Laura, Re Sartò Giulia (Sacco, Milano), Gambaro Giovanni, Ortalda Vittorio, Andreola Stefano (Verona Borgo Trento), Gesualdo Loreto, Di Palma Anna Maria, Cafiero Cesira, Ferrara Raffaella (Bari), La Manna Gaetano, Cianciolo Giuseppe, Zappulo Fulvia (Bologna), Lentini Paolo Luca, Fuso Valeria, Benedetti Claudia (Bassano del Grappa), Mallamaci Francesca, Panuccio Vincenzo (Reggio Calabria), Mancini Walter, Fabi Liana (Pordenone), Nordio Maurizio, Puggia Riccarda Maria (Treviso), Pani Antonello, Caria Stefania (Cagliari), Pinna Antonio Maria, Mereu Cristina, Patrizia Vatieri (Oristano), Santirosi Paola, Ciabattini Francesca (Foligno), Santoro Domenico, Gembillo Guido, Zirino Fortunata (Messina), Vezzoli Giuseppe, Quartagno Rita, Bologna Arianna, De Rosa Liliana (San Raffaele Milano), Zanella Monica, Mariotto Alice, Marchionna Nicola, Sgarabotto Luca (Vicenza).

Conflicts of Interest: The authors declare no conflict of interest.

References

1. Rodrıguez-Garcıa, M.; Gomez-Alonso, C.; Naves-Dıaz, M.; Diaz-Lopez, J.B.; Diaz-Corte, C.; Cannata-Andıa, J.B.; Asturias Study Group. Vascular calcifications, vertebral fractures and mortality in haemodialysis patients. *Nephrol. Dial. Transplant.* **2009**, *24*, 239–246. [CrossRef] [PubMed]
2. Ketteler, M.; Block, G.A.; Evenepoel, P.; Fukagawa, M.; Herzog, C.A.; McCann, L.; Moe, S.M.; Shroff, R.; Tonelli, M.A.; Toussaint, N.D.; et al. Executive summary of the 2017 KDIGO Chronic Kidney Disease-Mineral and Bone Disorder (CKD-MBD) Guideline Update: What's changed and why it matters. *Kidney Int.* **2017**, *92*, 26–36. [CrossRef] [PubMed]
3. Jono, S.; Shioi, A.; Ikari, Y.; Nishizawa, Y. Vascular calcification in chronic kidney disease. *J. Bone Miner. Metab.* **2006**, *24*, 176–181. [CrossRef] [PubMed]
4. Fusaro, M.; Gallieni, M.; Porta, C.; Nickolas, T.L.; Khairallah, P. Vitamin K effects in human health: New insights beyond bone and cardiovascular health. *J. Nephrol.* **2020**, *33*, 239–249. [CrossRef]
5. Fusaro, M.; Cianciolo, G.; Brandi, M.L.; Ferrari, S.; Nickolas, T.L.; Tripepi, G.; Plebani, M.; Zaninotto, M.; Iervasi, G.; La Manna, G.; et al. Vitamin K and Osteoporosis. *Nutrients* **2020**, *12*, 3625. [CrossRef] [PubMed] [PubMed Central]
6. Zebboudj, A.F.; Imura, M.; Bostrom, K. Matrix GLA protein, a regulatory protein for bone morphogenetic protein-2. *J. Biol. Chem.* **2002**, *277*, 4388–4394. [CrossRef]
7. Fusaro, M.; Giannini, S.; Gallieni, M.; Noale, M.; Tripepi, G.; Rossini, M.; Messa, P.; Rigotti, P.; Pati, T.; Barbisoni, F.; et al. Calcimimetic and vitamin D analog use inhemodialyzed patients is associated with increased levels of vitamin K dependent proteins. *Endocrine* **2016**, *51*, 333–341. [CrossRef]
8. Fusaro, M.; Mereu, M.C.; Aghi, A.; Iervasi, G.; Gallieni, M. Vitamin K and bone. *Clin. Cases Miner. Bone Metab.* **2017**, *14*, 200–206. [CrossRef] [PubMed] [PubMed Central]
9. Russo, D.; Tripepi, R.; Malberti, F.; Di Iorio, B.; Scognamiglio, B.; Di Lullo, L.; Paduano, I.G.; Tripepi, G.L.; Panuccio, V.A. Etelcalcetide in Patients on Hemodialysis with Severe Secondary Hyperparathyroidism. Multicenter Study in Real Life. *J. Clin. Med.* **2019**, *8*, 1066. [CrossRef]
10. Pasch, A.; Farese, S.; Gräber, S.; Wald, J.; Richtering, W.; Floege, J.; Jahnen-Dechent, W. Nanoparticle-based test measures overall propensity for calcification in serum. *J. Am. Soc. Nephrol.* **2012**, *23*, 1744–1752. [CrossRef] [PubMed] [PubMed Central]
11. Nakatani, S.; Mori, K.; Sonoda, M.; Nishide, K.; Uedono, H.; Tsuda, A.; Emoto, M.; Shoji, T. Association between Serum Zinc and Calcification Propensity (T_{50}) in Patients with Type 2 Diabetes Mellitus and In Vitro Effect of Exogenous Zinc on T_{50}. *Biomedicines* **2020**, *8*, 337. [CrossRef] [PubMed]
12. Takayama, Y.; Yasuda, Y.; Suzuki, S.; Shibata, Y.; Tatami, Y.; Shibata, K.; Niwa, M.; Sawai, A.; Morimoto, R.; Kato, S.; et al. Relationship between abdominal aortic and coronary artery calcification as detected by computed tomography in chronic kidney disease patients. *Heart Vessel.* **2016**, *31*, 1030–1037. [CrossRef] [PubMed]
13. Fusaro, M.; Schileo, E.; Crimi, G.; Aghi, A.; Bazzocchi, A.; Barbanti Brodano, G.; Girolami, M.; Sella, S.; Politi, C.; Ferrari, S.; et al. A Novel Quantitative Computer-Assisted Score Can Improve Repeatability in the Estimate of Vascular Calcifications at the Abdominal Aorta. *Nutrients* **2022**, *14*, 4276. [CrossRef] [PubMed] [PubMed Central]
14. Souberbielle, J.C.; Roth, H.; Fouque, D.P. Parathyroid hormone measurement in CKD. *Kidney Int.* **2010**, *77*, 93–100. [CrossRef] [PubMed]
15. Witteman, J.C.; Grobbee, D.E.; Valkenburg, H.A.; Stijnen, T.; Burger, H.; Hofman, A.; van Hemert, A.M. J-shaped relation between change in diastolic blood pressure and progression of aortic atherosclerosis. *Lancet* **1994**, *343*, 504–507. [CrossRef]

16. Genant, H.K.; Jergas, M.; Palermo, L.; Nevitt, M.; Valentin, R.S.; Black, D.; Cummings, S.R. Comparison of semiquantitative visual and quantitative morphometric assessment of prevalent and incident vertebral fractures in osteoporosis. *J. Bone Miner. Res.* **1996**, *11*, 984–996. [CrossRef]
17. Guglielmi, G.; Diacinti, D.; van Kuijk, C.; Aparisi, F.; Krestan, C.; Adams, J.E.; Link, T.M. Vertebral morphometry: Current methods and recent advances. *Eur. Radiol.* **2008**, *18*, 1484–1496. [CrossRef]
18. Fusaro, M.; Noale, M.; Viola, V.; Galli, F.; Tripepi, G.; Vajente, N.; Plebani, M.; Zaninotto, M.; Guglielmi, G.; Miotto, D.; et al. Vitamin K, Vertebral Fractures, Vascular Calcifications, and Mortality: VItamin K Italian (VIKI) Dialysis Study. *J. Bone Miner. Res.* **2012**, *27*, 2271–2278. [CrossRef]
19. Li, X.; Yu, L.; Asuncion, F.; Grisanti, M.; Alexander, S.; Hensley, K.; Han, C.-Y.; Niu, Q.-T.; Dwyer, D.; Villasenor, K.; et al. Etelcalcetide (AMG 416), a peptide agonist of the calcium-sensing receptor, preserved cortical bone structure and bone strength in subtotal nephrectomized rats with established secondary hyperparathyroidism. *Bone* **2017**, *105*, 163–172. [CrossRef]
20. Igarashi, S.; Kasukawa, Y.; Nozaka, K.; Tsuchie, H.; Abe, K.; Saito, H.; Shoji, R.; Kasama, F.; Harata, S.; Okamoto, K.; et al. Teriparatide and etelcalcetide improve bone, fibrosis, and fat parameters in chronic kidney disease model rats. *Osteoporos Sarcopenia* **2023**, *9*, 121–130. [CrossRef]
21. Khairallah, P.; Cherasard, J.; Sung, J.; Agarwal, S.; Aponte, M.A.; Bucovsky, M.; Fusaro, M.; Silberzweig, J.; Frumkin, G.N.; El Hachem, K.; et al. Changes in Bone Quality after Treatment with Etelcalcetide. *Clin. J. Am. Soc. Nephrol.* **2023**, *18*, 1456–1465. [CrossRef] [PubMed]
22. Wakamatsu, T.; Yamamoto, S.; Matsuo, K.; Taniguchi, M.; Hamano, T.; Fukagawa, M.; Kazama, J.J. Effectiveness of calcimimetics on fractures in dialysis patients with secondary hyperparathyroidism: Meta-analysis of randomized trials. *J. Bone Miner. Metab.* **2024**, *42*, 316–325. [CrossRef] [PubMed]
23. Palmer, S.C.; Mavridis, D.; Johnson, D.W.; Tonelli, M.; Ruospo, M.; Strippoli, G.F.M. Comparative Effectiveness of Calcimimetic Agents for Secondary Hyperparathyroidism in Adults: A Systematic Review and Network Meta-analysis. *Am. J. Kidney Dis.* **2020**, *76*, 321–330. [CrossRef] [PubMed]
24. Guo, Y.; Yang, X.; He, J.; Liu, J.; Yang, S.; Dong, H. Important roles of the Ca^{2+}-sensing receptor in vascular health and disease. *Life Sci.* **2018**, *209*, 217–227. [CrossRef] [PubMed]
25. Rodríguez, M.; Aguilera-Tejero, E.; Mendoza, F.J.; Guerrero, F.; López, I. Effects of calcimimetics on extraskeletal calcifications in chronic kidney disease. *Kidney Int. Suppl.* **2008**, *74*, S50–S54. [CrossRef] [PubMed]
26. Lopez, I.; Aguilera-Tejero, E.; Mendoza, F.J.; Almaden, Y.; Perez, J.; Martin, D.; Rodriguez, M. Calcimimetic R-568 decreases extraosseous calcifications in uremic rats treated with calcitriol. *J. Am. Soc. Nephrol.* **2006**, *17*, 795–804. [CrossRef]
27. Yu, L.; Tomlinson, J.E.; Alexander, S.T.; Hensley, K.; Han, C.-Y.; Dwyer, D.; Stolina, M.; Dean, C.; Goodman, W.G.; Richards, W.G.; et al. Etelcalcetide, A Novel Calcimimetic, Prevents Vascular Calcification in A Rat Model of Renal Insufficiency with Secondary Hyperparathyroidism. *Calcif. Tissue Int.* **2017**, *101*, 641–653. [CrossRef]
28. Colaianni, G.; Cuscito, C.; Mongelli, T.; Pignataro, P.; Buccoliero, C.; Liu, P.; Lu, P.; Sartini, L.; Di Comite, M.; Mori, G.; et al. The myokine irisin increases cortical bone mass. *Proc. Natl. Acad. Sci. USA* **2015**, *112*, 12157–12162, Erratum in *Proc. Natl. Acad. Sci. USA* **2015**, *112*, E5763. [CrossRef] [PubMed] [PubMed Central]
29. He, L.; He, W.Y.; Yang, W.L.; Zhang, A.H. Lower Serum Irisin Levels Are Associated with Increased Vascular Calcification in Hemodialysis Patients. *Kidney Blood Press. Res.* **2018**, *43*, 287–295. [CrossRef]

Journal of
Clinical Medicine

MDPI

Article

Contrast-Induced Nephropathy in Endovascular Patients: A Retrospective Cohort Study from a Vascular Surgery Clinic in Eastern Europe

Nicu Olariu [1], Felix-Mihai Maralescu [1,2,*], Flaviu Bob [1,2], Iulia Dana Grosu [1,2], Razvan Dragota-Pascota [1], Luciana Marc [1,2], Lazar Chisavu [1,2], Oana Albai [2,3], Ioana Adela Ratiu [4,5], Sorin Barac [6], Andreea Luciana Rață [6], Adelina Mzi [6] and Adelina Mihaescu [1,2]

1 Department of Internal Medicine II—Nephrology University Clinic, "Victor Babes" University of Medicine and Pharmacy, 300041 Timișoara, Romania; nicu.olariu@umft.ro (N.O.); bob.flaviu@umft.ro (F.B.); grosu.iulia@umft.ro (I.D.G.); razvan.dragota-pascota@umft.ro (R.D.-P.); marc.luciana@umft.ro (L.M.); chisavu.lazar@umft.ro (L.C.); mihaescu.adelina@umft.ro (A.M.)
2 Centre for Molecular Research in Nephrology and Vascular Disease, Faculty of Medicine, "Victor Babes" University of Medicine and Pharmacy, 300041 Timișoara, Romania; albai.oana@umft.ro
3 Department of Second Internal Medicine—Diabetes, Nutrition, Metabolic Diseases, and Systemic Rheumatology, "Victor Babes" University of Medicine and Pharmacy, 300041 Timisoara, Romania
4 Faculty of Medicine and Pharmacy, University of Oradea, 1st December Square 10, 410073 Oradea, Romania; ratiu_ioana@yahoo.com
5 Nephrology Department, Emergency Clinical Hospital Bihor County, 12 Corneliu Coposu Street, 410469 Oradea, Romania
6 Department of Vascular Surgery, Research Centre for Vascular and Endovascular Surgery, "Victor Babes" University of Medicine and Pharmacy, 300041 Timisoara, Romania; sorin.barac@umft.ro (S.B.); andreea.rata@umft.ro (A.L.R.); adelina.mzi@umft.ro (A.M.)
* Correspondence: mihai.maralescu@umft.ro

Abstract: Introduction: Contrast-induced nephropathy (CIN) has emerged as a prevalent and serious complication associated with the administration of iodinated contrast media during diagnostic and therapeutic procedures. Given the rising global prevalence of chronic kidney disease(CKD,) it is crucial to gain a deeper understanding of the risks linked to contrast media exposure. Therefore, the aim of this study, conducted at the Vascular Surgery Clinic in a tertiary hospital in Eastern Europe (Timisoara, Romania), is to assess the incidence of CIN and identify its associated risk factors among patients undergoing endovascular interventions. **Methods:** This retrospective cohort study was conducted using data from patients treated at a vascular surgery clinic in Timisoara, Romania, between 1 January 2018 and 31 December 2023. The study population included adult patients who underwent scheduled endovascular procedures and had serum creatinine measurements both before and after the procedure. **Results:** A total of 331 patients were included in the analysis (71.42% males with a mean age of 66.79 ± 9.86 years). In total, 9.22% of the patients had CKD, while 23.8% developed CIN. The mean age was significantly higher in the CIN group (68.4 years) compared to the non-CIN group (66.32 years) with a *p*-value of 0.093, indicating that older age is associated with a higher risk of CIN. A multivariate logistic regression analysis was performed to assess the association between various factors and the development of CIN. Higher hemoglobin levels were associated with reduced odds of CIN (OR = 0.792, 95% CI: 0.659–0.952, $p = 0.0148$), indicating that anemia is a significant risk factor for CIN, while CKD significantly increased the odds of CIN by 85.8% (OR = 1.858, 95% CI: 1.105–3.125, $p = 0.0023$), establishing CKD as a critical risk factor for CIN. **Conclusions:** While anemia and CKD were found to be significant predictors of CIN, further research on a wider population is required to validate these findings and explore additional risk factors. Our study shows that, in the context of elective endovascular procedures, addressing anemia correction and stabilizing creatinine levels to baseline represents a crucial strategy for reducing the risk of CIN.

Keywords: contrast-induced nephropathy; chronic kidney disease; endovascular procedures

1. Introduction

Acute kidney injury (AKI) is a significant clinical concern characterized by a rapid decline in renal function, often leading to adverse outcomes such as prolonged hospitalization, increased morbidity, and mortality. Among the various causes of AKI, contrast-induced nephropathy (CIN) has emerged as a prevalent and serious complication associated with the administration of iodinated contrast media during diagnostic and therapeutic procedures. The definition of CIN has been reported in many ways in the literature, being defined as an increase in serum creatinine levels of at least 0.5 mg/dL or a relative increase of 25% from baseline within 48 to 72 h following exposure to contrast agents [1,2]. Alternatively, as the acute kidney injury network (AKIN) Work Group states in the Kidney Disease: Improving Global Outcomes (KDIGO) AKI Guideline, there are no pathophysiological or epidemiological reasons why the definition and staging of CIN should differ from any other forms of AKI (increase in serum creatinine $\geq$0.3 mg/dL within 48 h, or $\geq$1.5 times baseline within 7 days or urine volume <0.5 mL/kg/h for 6 h) as per AKIN criteria [1,2]. This condition is particularly notable as it represents the third most common cause of hospital-acquired AKI, following decreased renal perfusion and nephrotoxic medications [3].

This risk is markedly heightened in individuals with chronic kidney disease (CKD), where the estimated glomerular filtration rate (eGFR) is less than 60 mL/min/1.73 m^2 [4]. The interplay between CIN and CKD is critical, as patients with CKD not only have a diminished renal reserve but also exhibit a higher susceptibility to nephrotoxic agents, including contrast media [5]. During endovascular procedures, particularly in patients with pre-existing renal impairment CIN can become a significant complication associated with the use of iodinated contrast media and the incidence in this patient population can be substantial, with studies indicating that it may affect up to 20% of individuals undergoing such interventions. The mechanisms underlying CIN in endovascular patients include renal vasoconstriction, hypoxia, and acute tubular necrosis, all of which can be exacerbated by the volume of contrast administered during procedures like endovascular aortic aneurysm repair [6,7]. Other studies show that the incidence of CIN can reach alarming rates in CKD patients undergoing procedures such as angiography or interventional radiology, with estimates suggesting that up to 50% of these patients may experience renal function deterioration post-contrast exposure and this highlights the necessity for careful risk assessment and management strategies tailored to this vulnerable population [8].

Diabetes mellitus (DM) is the most prevalent condition that significantly heightens the risk of developing CIN, particularly in patients with CKD undergoing endovascular procedures. Mechanisms linking DM and renal impairment are multifaceted, involving factors such as hyperglycemia, insulin resistance, and inflammation, which can lead to structural and functional changes in the kidneys [9]. Notably, individuals with diabetes are more likely to have coexisting conditions, such as hypertension and obesity, which further exacerbate the risk of renal injury following contrast exposure [10]. The bidirectional relationship between DM and CKD necessitates that healthcare providers prioritize early screening and intervention methods to mitigate the risk of CIN and its associated complications [11].

Strategies such as hydration, the use of alternative imaging modalities like carbon dioxide (CO_2) angiography, and the administration of nephroprotective agents (e.g., N-acetylcysteine and ascorbic acid) have been explored with encouraging outcomes [12]. Furthermore, recent guidelines emphasize the importance of individualized approaches based on the patient's renal function and overall health status [13].

Given the rising global prevalence of CKD, it is crucial to gain a deeper understanding of the risks linked to contrast media exposure. Therefore, the aim of this study, conducted at the Vascular Surgery Clinic in a tertiary hospital in Eastern Europe (Timisoara, Romania) is to assess the incidence of CIN and identify its associated risk factors among patients undergoing endovascular interventions.

2. Materials and Methods

2.1. Study Design and Population

This retrospective cohort study was conducted using data from patients treated at a vascular surgery clinic in Timisoara, Romania, between 1 January 2018 and 31 December 2023. The study population included adult patients who underwent scheduled endovascular procedures of the peripheral arteries (percutaneous angioplasty with or without stent insertion or diagnostic peripheral arteriopathy) and had serum creatinine measurements both before and after the procedure. Patients with elevated inflammatory marker values, sepsis, hemodynamically unstable, missing key data, and severe renal dysfunction (acute kidney injury at presentation or CKD stage 5 with eGFR < 15 mL/min at presentation) or those who did not have complete follow-up were excluded. The definition of CIN we used in this study was the one recommended by the KDIGO Guideline for AKI. Due to logistical reasons, we determined that a patient had CIN if there was an increase in serum creatinine of at least 0.3 mg/dL within 48 h after the administration of contrast media for the endovascular procedure. We could not measure timely urinary output or the change in baseline creatinine within 7 days. The contrast media used was either iopromid (low-osmolar, Ultravist 300 mg I/mL, produced by Bayer) or iodixanol (iso-osmolar, Visipaque 320 mg I/mL, produced by GE Healthcare) within the 50–150 mL range in quantity, infused intra-arterially. This study was conducted in accordance with the ethical principles outlined in the Declaration of Helsinki. The protocol was reviewed and approved by the hospital institutional ethics committee nr. 489/01.10.2024.

2.2. Data Collection

Data were extracted from patient medical records, including demographic characteristics (age, sex), medical history (CKD, DM, hypertension, ischemic heart disease, left ventricular hypertrophy (LVH) and heart failure), laboratory values (hemoglobin, serum creatinine at least 1 h before the procedure and 24–48 h after the procedure), and procedural details (type of procedure, contrast quantity, use of CIN prophylaxis) and their outcomes were evaluated in relation to the occurrence of CIN and other clinical variables. CIN was diagnosed as per AKIN group recommendations, as an increase of serum creatinine of at least 0.3 mg/dL within 48 h from the procedure.

2.3. Statistical Analysis

For descriptive analysis, continuous variables were summarized as means and standard deviations (SD), and categorical variables were expressed as counts and percentages. To compare baseline characteristics between patients with and without CIN, we used t-tests for normally distributed continuous variables, Mann–Whitney U tests for non-normally distributed continuous variables, and Chi-square tests or Fisher's exact tests (where appropriate) to compare categorical variables. For the primary analysis, Table 1 was generated to summarize patient characteristics stratified by the presence of CIN, and multivariate logistic regression analysis was performed to assess the association between various factors and the development of CIN. Statistical significance was determined using p-values, with a threshold set at 0.05.

Table 1. General values for the patients stratified by CIN.

	No CIN	CIN	*p*-Values
n	251	80	
Age (mean(SD))	66.3 (9.65)	68.44 (10.17)	0.093
Sex (%): f	67 (26.7)	26 (32.5)	0.388
m	184 (73.3)	54 (67.5)	
CKD (%): 0	236 (94.0)	64 (80.0)	<0.001
1	15 (6.0)	16 (20.0)	
DiabetesMelitus (%): 0	132 (52.6)	39 (48.8)	0.183
1	119 (47.4)	40 (50.0)	
Hypertension (%): 0	49 (19.5)	13 (16.2)	0.625
1	202 (80.5)	67 (83.8)	
LVH (%): 0	99 (39.4)	26 (32.9)	0.362
1	152 (60.6)	53 (67.1)	
Ischemic heart disease (%): 0	156 (62.2)	48 (60.8)	0.929
1	95 (37.8)	31 (39.2)	
Hearth failure (%): 0	113 (45.0)	33 (41.8)	0.706
1	138 (55.0)	46 (58.2)	
Hemoglobin (mean (SD))	13.32	12.35	<0.001
Serum Creatinine before procedure (mean (SD))	0.96 (0.24)	1.41 (0.52)	<0.001
Serum Creatinine within 48 h after procedure (mean (SD))	0.94 (0.26)	1.39 (0.62)	<0.0001
ContrastQuantity (mean (SD))	104.38 (24.51)	105.00 (30.40)	0.854

(1 = YES, 0 = NO).

2.4. Software

All statistical analyses were performed using RStudio 2024.04.2 + 764 for Windows, and visualizations were created using the ggplot2 package Version: 3.5.1. Table 1 was generated using the tableone package version 0.13.2, and the results were exported to Word documents using officer (version 0.6.7) and flextable (0.9.7) packages.

3. Results

A total of 331 patients were included in the analysis (71.42% male, and with a mean age of 66.79 ± 9.86 years). The prevalence of DM in the cohort was 47.9%; 9.22% of the patients had CKD, while 23.8% developed CIN. Other common comorbidities included hypertension (80.95%), ischemic heart disease (38.2%), and cardiac failure (55.2%). Table 1 provides a detailed summary of the demographic and clinical characteristics of the entire cohort divided by CIN status.

Moreover, 23.8% (n = 80) of the patients developed CIN. When assessed using the KDIGO criteria, all CIN patients exhibited Stage 1 AKI, characterized by a ≥0.3 mg/dL (≥26.5 µmol/L) increase in serum creatinine within 48 h or a 1.5–1.9-fold increase from baseline, without requiring renal replacement therapy. The mean age was not significantly higher in the CIN group (68.4) compared to the non-CIN group (66.30 years). The distribution of males and females is similar between the groups (73.3% male in the non-CIN group vs. 67.5% in the CIN group). The p-value of 0.338 suggests no significant difference in sex distribution between the groups. A significantly higher percentage of patients with CIN had CKD (20% in the CIN group vs. 6% in the non-CIN group). The p-value is <0.001, indicating a strong association between CKD and the development of CIN.

The prevalence of DM was slightly higher in the CIN group (50%) compared to the non-CIN group (47.4%), with a p-value of 0.183, suggesting a borderline association between diabetes and CIN. Hypertension was common in both groups (80.5 in the non-CIN group and 83.8% in the CIN group), with a p-value of 0.625, indicating no significant difference in the prevalence of hypertension between the groups. Slightly more patients with CIN had LVH (67.1%) compared to the non-CIN group (60.6%), with a p-value of 0.362. The amount of contrast used was similar between the groups (mean of 104.38 mL in the non-CIN group vs. 105.00 mL in the CIN group), with a p-value of 0.854, indicating no significant difference in contrast volume administration.

The prevalence of ischemic heart disease was similar in both groups (37.5% in the non-CIN group and 39.2% in the CIN group), with a p-value of 0.929, suggesting no significant association. On the other hand, more patients with CIN had heart failure (58.2%) compared to those without CIN (55.0%) with a p-value of 0.706, indicating no differences between them. The mean hemoglobin level was significantly lower in the CIN group (12.35 g/dL) compared to the non-CIN group (13.3 g/dL), with a p-value < 0.001, indicating a strong association between lower hemoglobin levels. The development of CIN suggests that patients with anemia are at a higher risk of developing CIN.

As expected, serum creatinine, before the procedure, was significantly higher in the CIN group (mean of 1.41 mg/dL) compared to the non-CIN group (0.96 mg/dL), with a p-value < 0.001, as depicted in Figures 1 and 2.

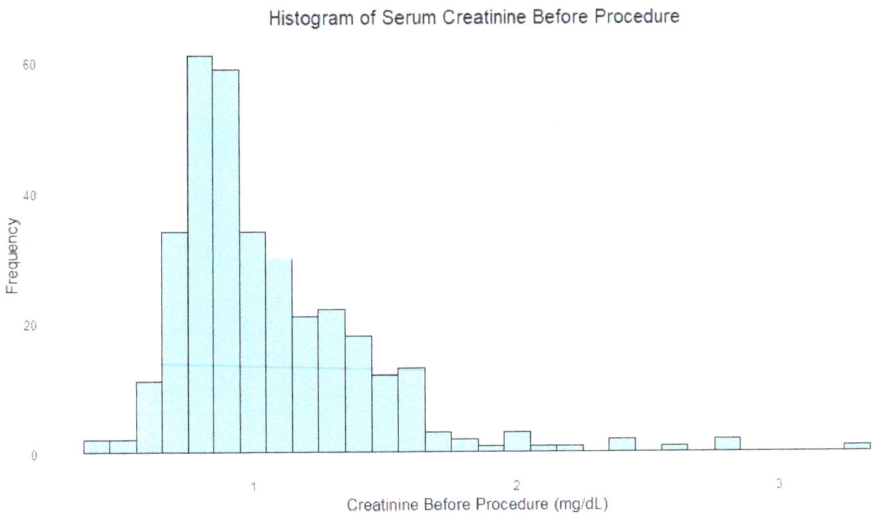

Figure 1. Histogram of serum creatinine before procedure.

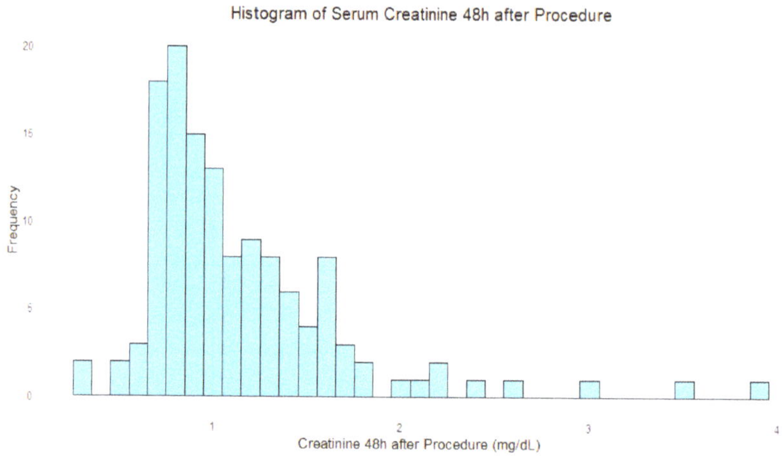

Figure 2. Histogram of serum creatinine 48 h after procedure.

A multivariate logistic regression analysis was performed to assess the association between various factors and the development of CIN. The model included age, hemoglobin, sex, CKD, diabetes mellitus, hypertension, ischemic heart disease, CIN prophylaxis, and heart failure as predictors. The results are as follows (Table 2).

Table 2. Multivariate logistic regression of factors associated with CIN.

Coefficients:	**Estimate**	**Std. Error**	**Z Value**	**Pr (>|z|)**
(Intercept)	−1.85514	2.01020	−0.923	0.3561
age	0.03670	0.02008	1.827	0.0677
Hemoglobin	−0.23311	0.09563	−2.438	0.0148 *
sexm	0.41376	0.41072	1.007	0.3137
CKD	0.61955	0.52478	1.181	0.0023 *
DiabetesMellitus	−0.23541	0.37930	−0.621	0.5348
Hypertension	−0.42109	0.52973	−0.795	0.4267
Ischemicheartdisease	−0.38200	0.40072	−0.953	0.3404
CINprophylaxy	0.19229	0.36340	0.529	0.5967
heartfailure	0.70939	0.46058	1.540	0.1235

* statistically significant.

The logistic regression model assessed predictors for contrast-induced nephropathy (CIN). The following results were obtained:

For every additional year of age, the odds of CIN increased by 3.74% (OR = 1.037, 95% CI: 0.997–1.079, $p = 0.0677$). This suggests that age might be a marginal predictor of CIN risk, although with no statistical significance, while higher hemoglobin levels were associated with reduced odds of CIN (OR = 0.792, 95% CI: 0.659–0.952, $p = 0.0148$), indicating that anemia is a significant risk factor for CIN.

CKD significantly increased the odds of CIN by 85.8% (OR = 1.858, 95% CI: 1.105–3.125, $p = 0.0023$), establishing CKD as a critical risk factor for CIN, while the presence of Diabetes Mellitus, hypertension, ischemic heart disease, heart failure, or even the CIN prophylaxis had no statistically significant impact on the risk of CIN prediction in our logistical regression model.

The performance of the logistic regression model was evaluated using a receiver operating characteristic (ROC) curve. The area under the curve (AUC) was 0.6934, indicating that the model has good discrimination in predicting the development of CIN (Figure 3).

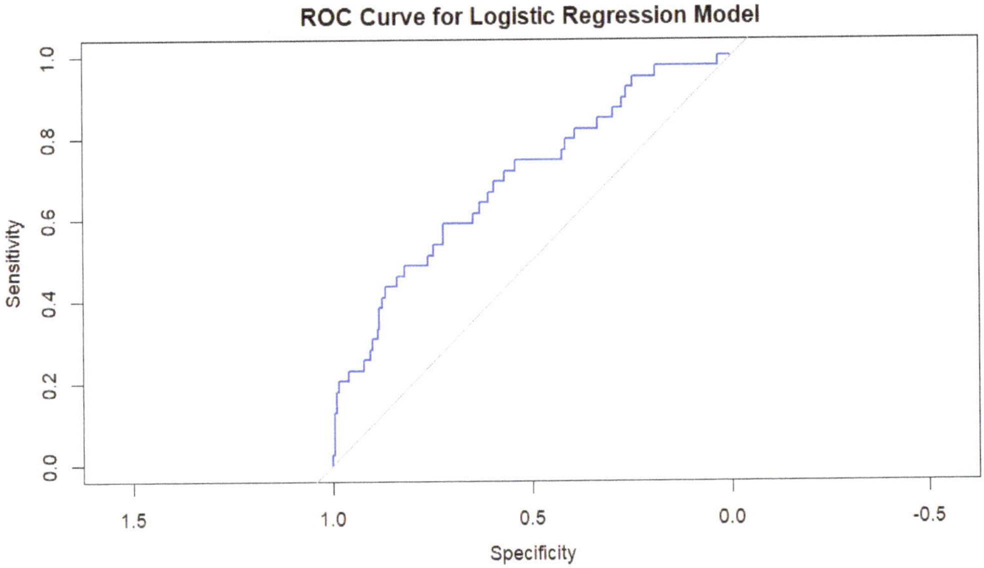

Figure 3. Roc curve for logistic regression model.

This interpretation highlights that the model is performing at a level that could be useful for clinical decision-making but also leaves space for refinement or the inclusion of additional predictive variables to improve accuracy.

To ensure the robustness of our predictive model and to avoid overfitting, we applied the Akaike Information Criterion (AIC) for stepwise selection. Using stepwise selection (both forward and backward elimination based on AIC), we iteratively removed variables that did not significantly improve the model fit. The AIC values for each step were recorded, and variables with the least contribution to the model were sequentially excluded. The final model retained the following predictors:

$$CIN \sim Age + Hemoglobin + Sex + Heart\ Failure$$

This model had the lowest AIC (232.4), indicating the best balance between explanatory power and simplicity. To assess the model's discrimination ability, we generated a receiver operating characteristic (ROC) curve, calculating the area under the curve (AUC) as a measure of predictive performance. The model's AUC was 0.69, suggesting good discrimination between patients who developed CIN and those who did not. Additionally, we assessed multicollinearity using variance inflation factors (VIFs), ensuring that no predictor exhibited substantial collinearity (VIF < 5 for all included variables), confirming the model's stability. These results indicate that age, hemoglobin, sex, and heart failure were the most critical independent predictors of CIN in our cohort, while other variables did not significantly improve model performance (Figure 4).

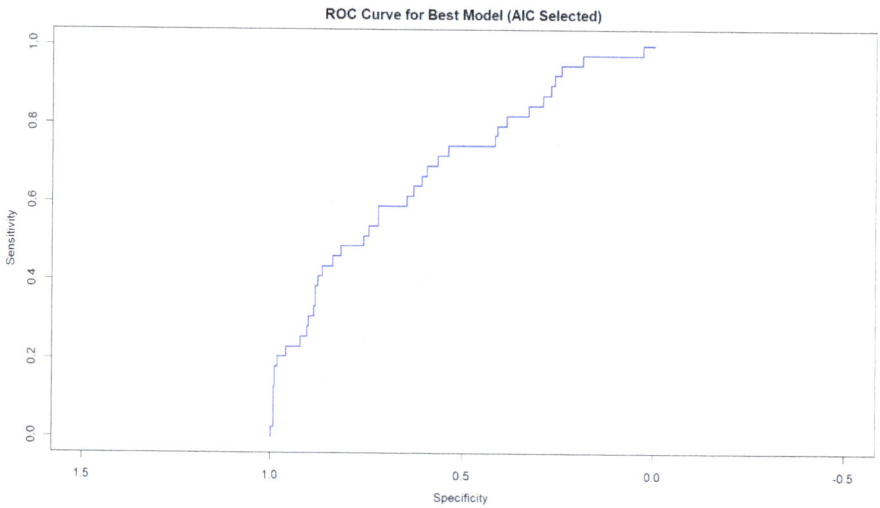

Figure 4. Roc curve for the best model (AIC selected).

4. Discussion

The discussion surrounding CIN in endovascular patients reveals a critical intersection of risk factors, particularly among older adults with diabetes, hypertension, cardiac failure, and especially anemic patients with concomitant CKD [14]. Our findings align with existing literature; however, from all the well-described risk factors, we found only hemoglobin levels and previous CKD as significant risk predictors for CIN. This could be the result of a homogeneous study population without acute diseases but with many chronic comorbidities. This heightened susceptibility can be attributed to multiple underlying mechanisms, including reduced renal reserve, pre-existing vascular complications, and physiological processes that exacerbate renal ischemia. Additionally, the cumulative impact of comorbidities further accelerates the decline in renal function [15,16].

Anemia has been recognized as a significant risk factor for the development of CIN, especially in patients undergoing procedures that involve the use of iodinated contrast media [17,18]. The interplay between anemia, aging processes, and CKD contributes to an increased susceptibility to CIN, highlighting the need for careful consideration in clinical practice. Numerous studies have indicated that reduced hemoglobin and hematocrit levels elevate the risk of CIN. For instance, research by Murakami et al. suggests that the deterioration of renal perfusion due to anemia may explain the heightened incidence of CIN in patients with low hematocrit and hemoglobin levels [14]. Additionally, Li et al. found that anemia serves as an independent predictor of CIN, with each 3% decrease in baseline hematocrit significantly increasing the likelihood of developing this condition [19]. Furthermore, the presence of CKD exacerbates the effects of anemia, as patients often exhibit lower hemoglobin levels due to decreased erythropoietin production and other factors related to kidney dysfunction [20]. In our study, despite the mild nature of anemia (with a mean hemoglobin level of 12.35 g/dL in the CIN group), its coexistence with microvascular alterations in CKD patients heightened the renal tubules' vulnerability to contrast-induced toxicity, ultimately contributing to the development of CIN.

The physiological changes that occur, including reduced renal blood flow and eGFR, make older adults more susceptible to the nephrotoxic effects of iodinated contrast agents [21]. Frailty in older patients often correlates with sarcopenia and decreased muscle mass, which can complicate the management of renal function and recovery following contrast exposure [22]. Older adults with CKD experience a higher prevalence of adverse outcomes, including prolonged hospitalization and increased mortality rates, particularly when undergoing procedures that require contrast media [23].

At the same time, this population is more likely to require contrast media, either for therapeutic purposes, such as endovascular procedures, or for diagnostic imaging enhanced by contrast agents, due to the accumulation of chronic diseases and comorbidities [19,24]. Therefore, it is imperative to adopt a comprehensive approach focusing on individualized risk assessment and the implementation of preventive measures to safeguard renal health during endovascular interventions.

In patients with heart failure, particularly those with reduced ejection fraction, the compromised cardiac output can lead to renal hypoperfusion, exacerbating the risk of CIN when iodinated contrast media is administered [25]. Conversely, CKD can contribute to the progression of heart failure by promoting fluid overload and increasing systemic vascular resistance, further complicating the management of both conditions [26]. DM is another critical risk factor for CIN, as it is often accompanied by microvascular complications that compromise renal function. The presence of DM not only increases the likelihood of developing CKD but also enhances the nephrotoxic effects of contrast media [16,27]. Published data indicate that diabetic patients are at a significantly greater risk of CIN, with estimates suggesting that up to 30% of individuals with diabetes may experience AKI following contrast exposure [27]. This relationship emphasizes the importance of vigilant screening and management of diabetic patients undergoing endovascular procedures, as well as the need for effective glycemic control to mitigate renal risks.

Despite a noticeably high number of patients with cardiac failure, hypertension, or DM, they were not proven to be significant risk factors for developing CIN. This may be explained by the fact that, in our cohort of patients, macrovascular complications prevailed, since it is well recognized in the literature that the more severe the microvascular diabetic complications, the less effectively endovascular procedures are and the more likely these types of patients require amputations. Another possible explanation could be related to the relatively low amount—a single administration—of contrast used in these procedures, with an average of 100 mL, while the risk of CIN increases with repeated doses [28], significantly beyond 150 mL, and continues to rise with every additional 100 mL, as suggested in recent CIN guidelines [29,30].

The interplay between the risk factors creates a multifaceted challenge in the management of patients undergoing endovascular procedures. The cumulative effect of these conditions can lead to a significant increase in the incidence of CIN, which is corroborated by our findings and the broader literature [15]. In this study, we identified several important predictors of CIN among patients undergoing endovascular procedures. Increasing age, anemia, and CKD were significantly associated with a higher risk of developing CIN, with older patients and those with CKD showing markedly elevated odds of developing this condition. Although other factors such as sex, diabetes mellitus, hypertension, ischemic heart disease, and heart failure were not found to be significant predictors in our multivariate model, CKD emerged as a strong and independent risk factor.

A key strength of our study is that it specifically focuses on CIN in patients undergoing peripheral endovascular procedures, where the amount of contrast media used is typically lower, and the patients tend to be more hemodynamically stable compared to those undergoing cardiac or neurovascular endovascular procedures. Additionally, none of the patients received repeated contrast administrations, which is another recognized risk factor for CIN [28,31–33]. This is because contrast-enhanced imaging, such as angio-CT, was performed prior to the intervention, and the endovascular procedures were scheduled electively, in a stable setting.

It Is worth noting that the mean "reat'Iine levels were not particularly elevated, indicating that these patients did not have advanced CKD, and none of them required dialysis during the study period. In summary, anemia, aging processes, and the presence of chronic kidney disease are critical factors that significantly increase the risk of developing CIN. The interplay between these elements underscores the necessity for vigilant monitoring and management of hemoglobin levels and renal function in at-risk populations to reduce the incidence of CIN. A limitation of this study is the relatively small sample size, which may impact the generalizability of the findings. Additionally, patients were not followed up for medium or long-term renal function outcomes after the episode of CIN (in those who developed it), limiting the understanding of its potential chronic effects.

5. Conclusions

Given the increasing global prevalence of CKD, a deeper understanding of the risks associated with contrast media exposure in this vulnerable population is essential for optimizing patient care and minimizing the potential for renal complications. While anemia and CKD were found to be significant predictors of CIN, further research on a wider population is required to validate these findings and explore additional risk factors. However, our study demonstrated that in the context of elective endovascular procedures, addressing anemia correction and stabilizing creatinine levels to baseline (preferably with a nephrologist consultation when available) represents a crucial strategy for reducing the risk of CIN.

Author Contributions: Conceptualization, N.O. and F.-M.M.; Data curation, F.-M.M., L.C., A.M. (Adelina Mzi) and A.M. (Adelina Mihaescu); Formal analysis, N.O., F.-M.M., L.M., L.C., O.A. and I.A.R.; Funding acquisition, I.A.R.; Investigation, F.-M.M., I.D.G., R.D.-P., L.M., S.B. and A.M. (Adelina Mihaescu); Methodology, F.-M.M., F.B. and A.L.R.; Project administration, A.M. (Adelina Mihaescu); Resources, I.D.G., L.M., L.C. and O.A.; Software, F.-M.M., R.D.-P. and S.B.; Supervision, F.B. and A.L.R.; Validation, A.L.R. and A.M. (Adelina Mihaescu); Visualization, N.O. and F.B.; Writing—original draft, N.O. and F.-M.M.; Writing—review and editing, N.O., F.-M.M. and A.M. (Adelina Mihaescu). All authors have read and agreed to the published version of the manuscript.

Funding: We would like to acknowledge VICTOR BABES UNIVERSITY OF MEDICINE AND PHARMACY TIMIȘOARA for their support in covering the costs of publication for this research paper.

Institutional Review Board Statement: The study was conducted in accordance with the Declaration of Helsinki, and approved by the Institutional Review Board (or Ethics Committee) of The Decision of the Local Scientific Research Ethics Committee of the "Pius Brînzeu" County Emergency Clinical Hospital Timișoara Nr. 489/01.10.2024.

Informed Consent Statement: Informed consent was obtained from all subjects involved in the study.

Data Availability Statement: The datasets analyzed during the current study are available from the corresponding author upon reasonable request.

Conflicts of Interest: The authors declare no conflicts of interest.

References

1. Ali, A.; Bhan, C.; Malik, M.B.; Ahmad, M.Q.; Sami, S.A. The Prevention and Management of Contrast-induced Acute Kidney Injury: A Mini-review of the Literature. *Cureus* **2018**, *10*, e3284. [CrossRef] [PubMed]
2. Andreucci, M.; Faga, T.; Pisani, A.; Sabbatini, M.; Russo, D.; Michael, A. Prevention of contrast-induced nephropathy through a knowledge of its pathogenesis and risk factors. *Sci. World J.* **2014**, *2014*, 823169. [CrossRef]
3. Kidney Disease: Improving Global Outcomes (KDIGO) Acute Kidney Injury Work Group. KDIGO Clinical Practice Guideline for Acute Kidney Injury. *Kidney Int. Suppl.* **2012**, *2*, 1–138.
4. Mohammed, N.M.A.; Mahfouz, A.; Achkar, K.; Rafie, I.; Hajar, R. Contrast-induced nephropathy. *Heart Views* **2013**, *14*, 106. [CrossRef] [PubMed]

5. Kaliyaperumal, Y.; Sivadasan, S.; Aiyalu, R. Contrast-Induced Nephropathy: An Overview. *Dr Sulaiman Al Habib Med. J.* **2023**, *5*, 118–127. [CrossRef]
6. Saratzis, A.N.; Goodyear, S.; Sur, H.; Saedon, M.; Imray, C.; Mahmood, A. Acute Kidney Injury After Endovascular Repair of Abdominal Aortic Aneurysm. *J. Endovasc. Ther.* **2013**, *20*, 315–330. [CrossRef] [PubMed]
7. Katsiki, N.; Athyros, V.G.; Karagiannis, A.; Mikhailidis, D.P. Contrast-induced nephropathy: An "all or none" phenomenon? *Angiology* **2015**, *66*, 508–513. [CrossRef]
8. Delgado Acosta, F.; Jiménez Gómez, E.; Bravo Rey, I.; Valverde Moyano, R.; de Asís Bravo-Rodriguez, F.; Oteros Fernández, R. Contrast-induced nephropathy: A dilemma between loss of neurons or nephrons in the setting of endovascular treatment of acute ischemic stroke. *Int. Neuroradiol.* **2020**, *26*, 33–37. [CrossRef] [PubMed]
9. Schrauben, S.J.; Chen, H.Y.; Lin, E.; Jepson, C.; Yang, W.; Scialla, J.J.; Fischer, M.J.; Lash, J.P.; Fink, J.C.; Hamm, L.L.; et al. Hospitalizations among adults with chronic kidney disease in the United States: A cohort study. *PLoS Med.* **2020**, *17*, e1003470. [CrossRef] [PubMed]
10. Murphy, D.; McCulloch, C.E.; Lin, F.; Banerjee, T.; Bragg-Gresham, J.L.; Eberhardt, M.S.; Morgenstern, H.; Pavkov, M.E.; Saran, R.; Powe, N.R.; et al. Trends in prevalence of chronic kidney disease in the United States. *Ann. Intern. Med.* **2016**, *165*, 473–481. [CrossRef]
11. Afkarian, M.; Sachs, M.C.; Kestenbaum, B.; Hirsch, I.B.; Tuttle, K.R.; Himmelfarb, J.; de Boer, I.H. Kidney disease and increased mortality risk in type 2 diabetes. *J. Am. Soc. Nephrol.* **2013**, *24*, 302–308. [CrossRef] [PubMed]
12. Rollins, K.; Noorani, A.; Janeckova, L.; Jones, T.; Griffiths, M.; Baker, M.P.; Boyle, J.R. Ascorbic acid ameliorates renal injury in a murine model of contrast-induced nephropathy. *BMC Nephrol.* **2017**, *18*, 1–9. [CrossRef] [PubMed]
13. Palli, E.; Makris, D.; Papanikolaou, J.; Garoufalis, G.; Tsilioni, I.; Zygoulis, P.; Zakynthinos, E. The impact of N-acetylcysteine and ascorbic acid in contrast-induced nephropathy in critical care patients: An open-label randomized controlled study. *Crit. Care* **2017**, *21*, 1–9. [CrossRef]
14. Murakami, R.; Kumita, S.I.; Hayashi, H.; Sugizaki, K.I.; Okazaki, E.; Kiriyama, T.; Hakozaki, K.; Tani, H.; Miki, I.; Takeda, M. Anemia and the risk of contrast-induced nephropathy in patients with renal insufficiency undergoing contrast-enhanced MDCT. *Eur. J. Radiol.* **2013**, *82*, e521–e524. [CrossRef] [PubMed]
15. Dinku, B.; Hailu, H.E.; Girma, B. Prevalence and Associated Factors of Chronic Kidney Disease among Diabetic and Hypertensive Patients at Ambo Town Public Hospitals of West Shewa Zone, Oromia Region, Ethiopia. *J. Nephrol. Endocrinol. Res.* **2022**, 1–5. Available online: https://www.onlinescientificresearch.com/articles/prevalence-and-associated-factors-of-chronic-kidney-disease-among-diabetic-and-hypertensive-patients-at-ambo-town-public-hospitals.pdf (accessed on 30 January 2025). [CrossRef]
16. Hussain, S.; Habib, A.; Najmi, A.K. Limited knowledge of chronic kidney disease among type 2 diabetes mellitus patients in India. *Int. J. Environ. Res. Public Health* **2019**, *16*, 1443. [CrossRef] [PubMed]
17. Liang, W.; Yu, C.J.; Wang, Q.Y.; Yu, J. Anemia is associated with increased risk of contrast-induced acute kidney injury: A Systematic Review and Meta-analysis. *Bioengineered* **2021**, *12*, 648–661. [CrossRef]
18. Stauder, R.; Thein, S.L. Anemia in the elderly: Clinical implications and new therapeutic concepts. *Haematologica* **2014**, *99*, 1127–1130. [CrossRef] [PubMed]
19. Li, W.H.; Li, D.Y.; Han, F.; Xu, T.D.; Zhang, Y.B.; Zhu, H. Impact of anemia on contrast-induced nephropathy (CIN) in patients undergoing percutaneous coronary interventions. *Int. Urol. Nephrol.* **2013**, *45*, 1065–1070. [CrossRef] [PubMed]
20. Demircelik, M.B.; Kurtul, A.; Ocek, H.; Cakmak, M.; Ureyen, C.; Eryonucu, B. Association between platelet-to-lymphocyte ratio and contrast-induced nephropathy in patients undergoing percutaneous coronary intervention for acute coronary syndrome. *Cardiorenal Med.* **2015**, *5*, 96–104. [CrossRef] [PubMed]
21. Han, P.; Yu, H.; Ma, Y.; Kang, L.; Fu, L.; Jia, L.; Chen, X.; Yu, X.; Hou, L.; Wang, L.; et al. The increased risk of sarcopenia in patients with cardiovascular risk factors in Suburb-Dwelling older Chinese using the AWGS definition. *Sci. Rep.* **2017**, *7*, 9592. [CrossRef] [PubMed]
22. Formiga, F.; Moreno-González, R.; Corsonello, A.; Carlsson, A.; Ärnlöv, J.; Mattace-Raso, F.; Kostka, T.; Weingart, C.; Roller-Wirnsberger, R.; Tap, L.; et al. Diabetes, sarcopenia and chronic kidney disease; the Screening for CKD among Older People across Europe (SCOPE) study. *BMC Geriatr.* **2022**, *22*, 254. [CrossRef]
23. Artzi-Medvedik, R.; Kob, R.; Fabbietti, P.; Lattanzio, F.; Corsonello, A.; Melzer, Y.; Roller-Wirnsberger, R.; Wirnsberger, G.; Mattace-Raso, F.; Tap, L.; et al. Impaired kidney function is associated with lower quality of life among community-dwelling older adults. *BMC Geriatr.* **2020**, *20*, 1–10. [CrossRef]
24. Ran, L.; Wang, L.; Cai, T. Impact of Sarcopenia on Prognosis in Frail Elderly Patients with Chronic Kidney Disease. *Proc. Anticancer Res.* **2023**, *7*, 35–40. Available online: http://ojs.bbwpublisher.com/index.php/PAR (accessed on 30 January 2025).
25. Iida, H.; Hanaoka, H.; Okada, Y.; Kiyokawa, T.; Takakuwa, Y.; Yamada, H.; Okazaki, T.; Ozaki, S.; Yamaguchi, K.; Nakajima, Y.; et al. A low perfusion-metabolic mismatch in 99mTl and 123I-BMIPP scintigraphy predicts poor prognosis in systemic sclerosis patients with asymptomatic cardiac involvement. *Int. J. Rheum. Dis.* **2019**, *22*, 1008–1015. [CrossRef] [PubMed]

26. Taylor, R.S.; Dalal, H.M.; Zwisler, A.D. Cardiac rehabilitation for heart failure: "Cinderella" or evidence-based pillar of care? *Eur. Heart J.* **2023**, *44*, 1511–1518. [CrossRef] [PubMed]
27. Fiseha, T. Prevalence of Chronic Kidney Disease and Associated Risk Factors among Diabetic Patients in Southern Ethiopia. *Am. J. Health Res.* **2014**, *2*, 216. [CrossRef]
28. Dinesch, V.; Dinesch, M.; Macarie, C.; Sirbu, I.V.; Buruian, M. Risk of Contrast-Induced Nephropathy after Repeated Contrast Medium Administration. *Acta Med. Marisiensis* **2018**, *64*, 108–110. [CrossRef]
29. ACR Manual on Contrast Media. 2024 ACR Committee on Drugs and Contrast Media. 2024. Available online: https://www.acr.org/Clinical-Resources/Clinical-Tools-and-Reference/Contrast-Manual (accessed on 30 January 2025).
30. Mullasari, A.; Victor, S.M. Victor Update on contrast induced nephropathy. *ESC Counc. Cardiol. Pract.* **2014**, *4*, 13.
31. Cichoń, M.; Wybraniec, M.T.; Okoń, O.; Zielonka, M.; Antoniuk, S.; Szatan, T.; Mizia-Stec, K. Repeated Dose of Contrast Media and the Risk of Contrast-Induced Acute Kidney Injury in a Broad Population of Patients Hospitalized in Cardiology Department. *J. Clin. Med.* **2023**, *12*, 2166. [CrossRef]
32. Sudarski, D.; Naami, R.; Shehadeh, F.; Elias, A.; Kerner, A.; Aronson, D. Risk of worsening renal function following repeated exposures to contrast media during percutaneous coronary interventions. *J. Am. Heart Assoc.* **2021**, *10*, e021473. [CrossRef] [PubMed]
33. Betoko, A.; Matheson, M.B.; Ostovaneh, M.R.; Miller, J.M.; Brinker, J.; Cox, C.; Lima, J.A.; Arbab-Zadeh, A. Acute Kidney Injury After Repeated Exposure to Contrast Material for Coronary Angiography. *Mayo Clin Proc. Innov. Qual. Outcomes* **2021**, *5*, 46–54. [CrossRef] [PubMed]

Journal of
Clinical Medicine

MDPI

Article

Pediatric Chronic Kidney Disease During Pandemic Conditions—A Single-Center Experience

Łukasz Biesiadecki [1], Joanna Jacuńska [1], Paulina Tomecka [1], Aleksandra Bruciak [1] and Kinga Musiał [2,*]

1 Students' Scientific Association, Department of Pediatric Nephrology, Wroclaw Medical University, Borowska 213, 50-556 Wroclaw, Poland
2 Department of Pediatric Nephrology, Wroclaw Medical University, Borowska 213, 50-556 Wroclaw, Poland
* Correspondence: kinga.musial@umw.edu.pl; Tel.: +48-71-736-44-70

Abstract: Background/Objectives: The prevalence of chronic kidney disease (CKD) is increasing worldwide, and this tendency is also visible in pediatric patients. The major clinical challenge is to achieve a diagnosis as early as possible, despite an overt clinical course, especially in the early stages of the disease. Unfavorable external conditions may disturb the proper treatment of chronically ill patients and delay the time of diagnosis. The recent COVID-19 pandemia might have altered the usual diagnostic pathways of different comorbidities, and CKD was probably one of them. However, there are no data on newly diagnosed CKD in children during the time of the pandemia, so our aim was to approach this problem. **Methods**: We analyzed medical records of 154 children with CKD who were hospitalized in the Department of Pediatric Nephrology in prepandemic (years 2015–2019) vs. pandemic and postpandemic (2020–2024) conditions, analyzing the eGFR value and stage of CKD at diagnosis, the underlying diseases leading to CKD, and sex-related differences. **Results**: The number of patients who were diagnosed with CKD in both time periods was comparable. Children hospitalized in the years 2020–2024 presented more often with advanced stages of CKD. The trend towards an increasing share of glomerulopathies, acute kidney injury, and unknown causes of CKD was noticeable under pandemic conditions. **Conclusions**: The COVID-19 pandemic could, probably owing to reduced access to primary healthcare and disrupted routine check-ups, delay the process of diagnosing CKD in children.

Keywords: chronic kidney disease (CKD); congenital anomalies of the kidney and urinary tract (CAKUT); COVID-19; glomerulopathies

1. Introduction

The epidemiological assessment of chronic kidney disease (CKD) in children faces two significant challenges. First, there is a paucity of data on the epidemiology of early-stage CKD in the pediatric population, as the condition often progresses asymptomatically, contributing to under-reporting and underdiagnosis in the primary care setting [1]. Second, the clinically silent progression of renal function decline may delay the moment of placing the patient in nephrological care, thus overlooking aggravation to the advanced stages of CKD.

The problem becomes more serious when the numbers are examined. According to data from several European pediatric nephrology societies, the prevalence of early-stage CKD is estimated to be approximately 11–12 cases per million age-related population (pmarp) for stages 3–5 and 8 pmarp for stages 4–5 [2]. A few population-based studies suggest that the prevalence of all-stage CKD in the pediatric population may be as high as

1% [3]. Moreover, the overall incidence of CKD among children has shown an increasing trend for the last 30 years [4].

According to various registries, 40–62% of childhood CKD are due to congenital anomalies of the kidneys and urinary tract (CAKUT) [2,5]. The percentage of candidates whose primary cause of kidney disease is CAKUT has been steadily increasing during a 10-year observation period [6].

The abovementioned trends could have been modified, or even aggravated, by the recent COVID-19 burden, yet there are no publications concerning the impact of pandemic conditions on the CKD epidemiology.

Therefore, our aim was to analyze retrospectively the epidemiology of CKD in children in the last 10 years, taking into account multiple variables at diagnosis: age, kidney function and CKD stage, causative factors of CKD, and sex-related differences, with special focus on the pandemic conditions and their potential influence on CKD in the pediatric population.

2. Material and Methods

The medical records of 154 pediatric patients with newly diagnosed chronic kidney disease, hospitalized at the Department of Pediatric Nephrology between 2015 and 2024, were retrospectively analyzed. Patients were stratified into two groups based on the time of diagnosis: prepandemic (2015–2019) and pandemic/postpandemic (2020–2024). Medical records were evaluated for age, gender, CKD stage at diagnosis, and CKD etiology, with comparisons being made between the two timeframes.

The basic demographic data of the studied population are presented in Table 1.

Table 1. Basic demographic data of patients with chronic kidney disease (CKD).

	2015–2019	2020–2024
Number of all CKD patients	74	79
Males %	59	62
Females %	41	38
Number of patients ≤ 2 years old	27	23
Males %	63	57
Females %	37	43
Number of patients > 2 years old	47	56
Males %	57	64
Females %	43	36

CKD was defined according to the Kidney Disease Outcomes Quality Initiative (KDIGO) guidelines, as either structural or functional kidney damage persisting for at least three months or a reduction in estimated glomerular filtration rate (eGFR) to below 60 mL/min/1.73 m^2 in children older than two years [5]. CKD was classified into five stages based on the degree of kidney function impairment: stage 1 CKD—eGFR $\geq$ 90 mL/min/1.73 m^2; stage 2—eGFR 60–89 mL/min/1.73 m^2; stage 3—eGFR 30–59 mL/min/1.73 m^2; stage 4—eGFR 15–29 mL/min/1.73 m^2; and stage 5—eGFR < 15 mL/min/1.73 m^2 (Table 2). For children under two years of age, with eGFR values physiologically below 60 mL/min/1.73 m^2, a CKD diagnosis was made based on the serum creatinine concentration, adjusted to the age-specific reference values. The eGFR values were calculated based on the Schwartz formula [7].

Table 2. Proportions of patients with CKD stages 1–5 at diagnosis in years 2015–2019 and 2020–2024.

	2015–2019	2020–2024
Number of patients > 2 years old	47	56
Median eGFR [ml/min/1.73 m^2] (IQR)	73 (50–91)	42 (22–99) #
Children with CKD stage 1 [%]	28	26
Children with CKD stage 2 [%]	36	16
Children with CKD stage 3 [%]	17	21
Children with CKD stage 4 [%]	13	20
Children with CKD stage 5 [%]	6	16

CKD—chronic kidney disease; eGFR—estimated glomerular filtration rate; IQR—interquartile range; # $p < 0.05$ Mann–Whitney U test.

The statistical analysis was performed using Statistica ver. 13 (StatSoft, Tulsa, OK, USA). The chi-square test and Fisher's exact test were employed to assess the significance of differences between categories. Continuous variables were compared with the use of a non-parametric Mann–Whitney U-test. A p-value < 0.05 was considered statistically significant.

3. Results

3.1. CKD Stage Distribution and eGFR Trends at Diagnosis

The numbers of newly diagnosed CKD patients within the prepandemic (2015–2019) and pandemic/postpandemic (2020–2024) periods were comparable (Table 2). The distribution of CKD stages at diagnosis across these two periods showed no statistically significant difference (Figure 1). However, when stratified according to the eGFR values of < and ≥60 mL/min/1.73 m^2, there was a statistically significant shift towards the advanced stages of CKD at diagnosis within the 2020–2024 period (Figure 2).

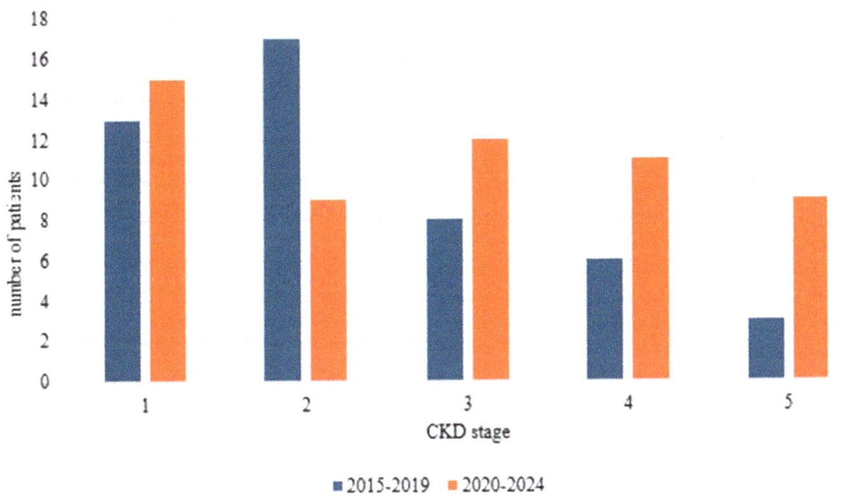

Figure 1. CKD stage at diagnosis in years 2015–2019 and 2020–2024; χ^2 test $p = 0.13$; CKD—chronic kidney disease.

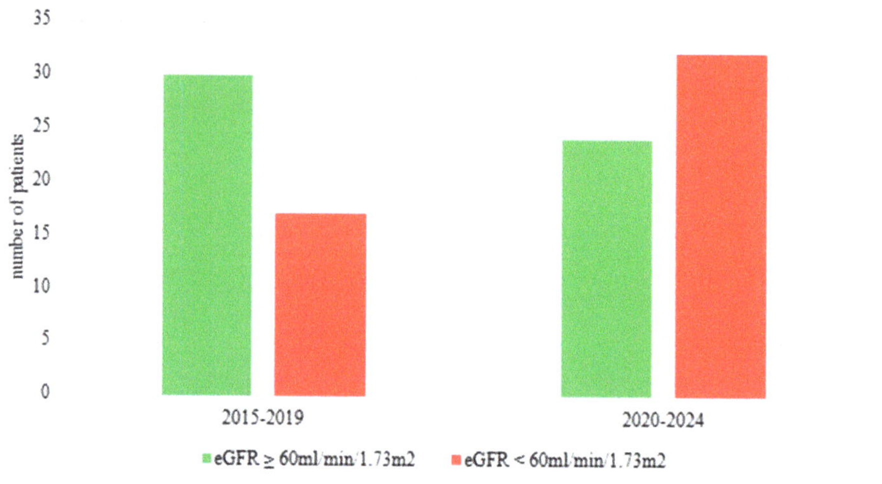

Figure 2. Proportions of patients with mild CKD (eGFR $\geq$ 60 mL/min/1.73 m^2) and advanced CKD (eGFR < 60 mL/min/1.73 m^2) at diagnosis in years 2015–2019 and 2020–2024; χ^2 test $p = 0.03$; eGFR—estimated glomerular filtration rate; CKD—chronic kidney disease.

3.2. Sex Differences in CKD Population at Diagnosis

There was a trend towards earlier diagnoses of CKD in males (CKD stage 1–2) and a slightly higher proportion of females were diagnosed in the advanced CKD stage (mainly stage 5), but these borderline differences missed statistical significance (Figure 3).

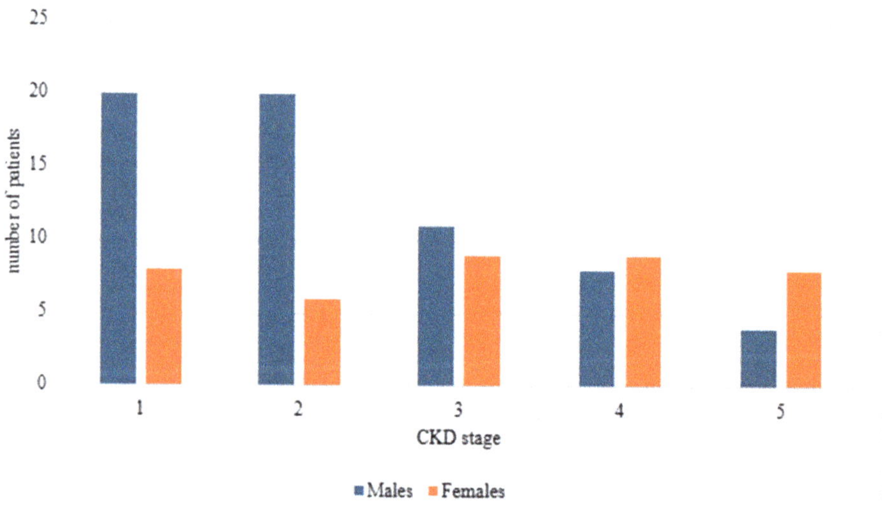

Figure 3. CKD stage at diagnosis in reference to gender in years 2015–2024; χ^2 test $p = 0.05$; CKD—chronic kidney disease.

However, the analysis of sex in relation to CKD severity, stratified as mild (eGFR < 60 mL/min/1.73 m^2) or advanced (eGFR $\geq$ 60 mL/min/1.73 m^2), revealed the dominance of males among patients with mild CKD and a higher proportion of females with advanced CKD (Figure 4). This sex-based difference reached statistical significance ($p = 0.004$).

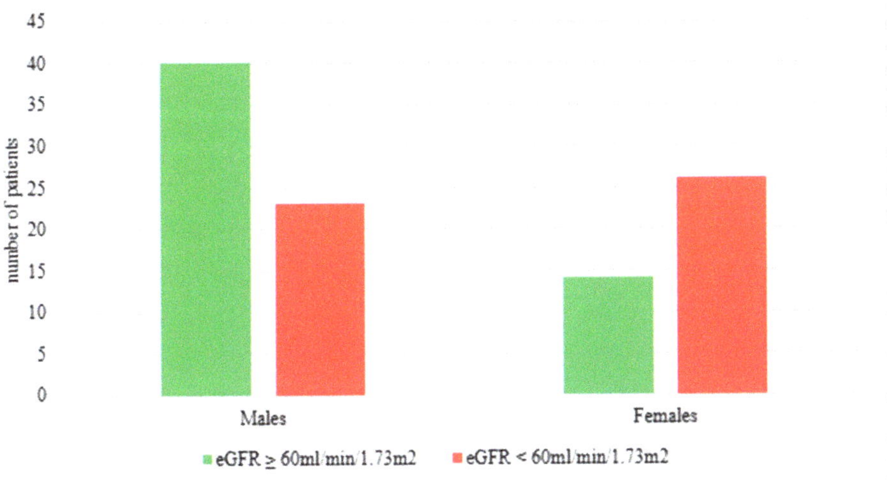

Figure 4. Proportions of males and females with early CKD (eGFR $\geq$ 60 mL/min/1.73 m^2) and advanced CKD (eGFR < 60 mL/min/1.73 m^2) at diagnosis in years 2015–2024; χ^2 test $p = 0.004$; eGFR—estimated glomerular filtration rate; CKD—chronic kidney disease.

3.3. Etiology of CKD in Relation to Age

The proportions of various diseases contributing to the CKD etiology remained similar within the age groups analyzed in the periods of 2015–2019 vs. 2020–2024. In children who were ≤2 years old, CAKUT was the dominant causative factor both before and during/after COVID-19, with a strong prevalence over AKI, genetic, and unknown causes (Table 3). In patients who were >2 years old, CAKUT remained responsible for less than half of CKD cases, whereas AKI, glomerulopathies, and unknown causes increased their shares compared to younger patients, irrespective of the analyzed time period. However, the presence of single-patient representatives in certain categories made the interpretation of these results rather difficult.

Table 3. Etiology of chronic kidney disease (CKD) in pre- and pandemic/postpandemic conditions according to the patients' age.

	2015–2019	2020–2024
Patients ≤ 2 years old [N]	27	23
CAKUT [N/%]	20/75	19/84
AKI [N/%]	2/7	2/8
Genetic [N/%]	3/11	1/4
Unknown [N/%]	2/7	1/4
Patients > 2 years old [N]	47	56
CAKUT [N/%]	22/47	27/48
AKI [N/%]	4/9	5/9
Genetic [N/%]	3/6	4/7
GN [N/%]	3/6	8/14.5
Neoplastic [N/%]	3/6	3/5
SD [N/%]	5/11	1/2
Unknown [N/%]	7/15	8/14.5

CAKUT—congenital anomalies of the kidney and urinary tract; AKI—acute kidney injury; GN—glomerulopathy; SD—systemic disease.

Therefore, we compared the entire group of children who were diagnosed within the first 2 years of life with those who were diagnosed at an older age in order to examine the age-related discrepancies (Figure 5). In patients who were ≤2 years of age, CAKUT was the most prevalent cause, accounting for 80% of cases. In patients who were >2 years, CAKUT remained the leading cause, but decreased to 48% at the expense of growing incidences of glomerulopathies, systemic diseases, and unknown causes of CKD (Figure 5).

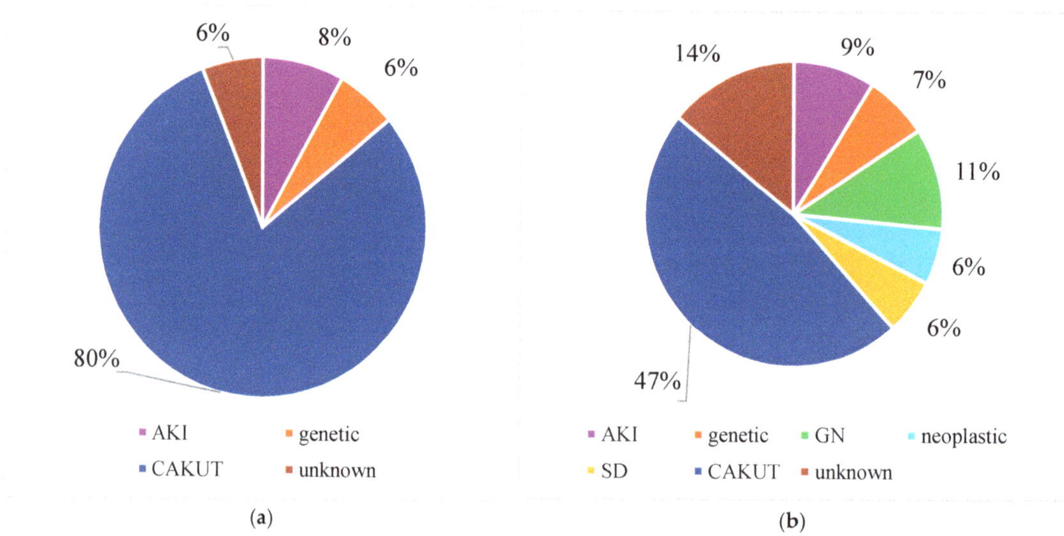

Figure 5. (**a**) CKD etiology in patients aged ≤ 2 years at diagnosis in 2015–2024 period; (**b**) CKD etiology in patients aged > 2 years at diagnosis in 2015–2024 period; CKD—chronic kidney disease; AKI—acute kidney injury; GN—glomerulopathy; SD—systemic disease; CAKUT—congenital anomalies of the kidney and urinary tract.

3.4. Etiology of CKD in Relation to Sex

CAKUT was the leading etiology of CKD in both analyzed periods and irrespective of sex (Table 4).

In the years 2015–2019, the higher incidence of CAKUT was related to the male sex of patients, but this trend did not endure during the 2020–2024 period (Table 4). Meanwhile, the proportion of genetic disorders seemed higher in females in both periods (Table 4), but these differences were again difficult to interpret due to the possible bias related to the small numbers of patients (Figure 6).

Table 4. Etiology of chronic kidney disease (CKD) in pre- and pandemic/postpandemic conditions according to the patients' gender.

	2015–2019	2020–2024
Females [N]	30	30
CAKUT [N/%]	15/50	17/57
AKI [N/%]	2/7	3/10
Genetic [N/%]	2/7	2/7
GN [N/%]	4/13	2/7
Neoplastic [N/%]	1/3	1/3
SD [N/%]	3/10	0
Unknown [N/%]	3/10	5/16

Table 4. *Cont.*

	2015–2019	2020–2024
Males [N]	44	49
CAKUT [N/%]	28/64	29/59
AKI [N/%]	4/9	4/8
Genetic [N/%]	½	3/6
GN [N/%]	½	6/13
Neoplastic [N/%]	2/5	2/4
SD [N/%]	2/5	½
Unknown [N/%]	6/13	4/8

CAKUT—congenital anomalies of the kidney and urinary tract; AKI—acute kidney injury; GN—glomerulopathy; SD—systemic disease.

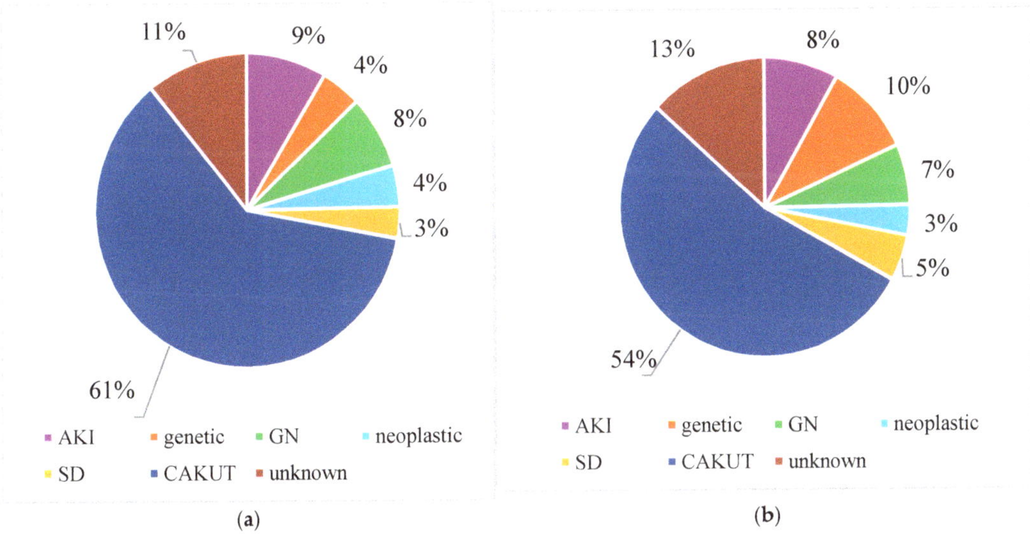

Figure 6. (**a**) CKD etiology in males in 2015–2024 period; (**b**) CKD etiology in females in 2015–2024 period; CKD—chronic kidney disease; AKI—acute kidney injury; GN—glomerulopathy; SD—systemic disease; CAKUT—congenital anomalies of the kidney and urinary tract.

3.5. Etiology of CKD in Relation to the Severity of the Disease

In the pre-COVID-19 era, the number of patients with CKD stage 1–2 at diagnosis exceeded that of children with CKD stage 3–5, whereas in the pandemic and postpandemic periods, the majority of newly diagnosed children with CKD presented with advanced CKD (Table 5).

The etiology of mild and advanced pediatric CKD at our center has shown a distinct shift between the 2015–2019 and 2020–2024 periods. In mild CKD (eGFR $\geq$ 60 mL/min/1.73 m^2), CAKUT remained the most common cause, accounting for nearly half of the cases in the years 2015–2019 and more than a half in the years 2020–2024 (Table 5). A similar increasing trend was found for glomerulopathies (Table 5). When the 2015–2024 period was analyzed as a whole, CAKUT as a main causative factor was followed by cases of unknown origin and glomerulopathies (Figure 7).

In advanced CKD (eGFR < 60 mL/min/1.73 m^2), the proportion of CAKUT cases decreased in both the pre- and postpandemic periods, mainly at the cost of increasing numbers of unknown etiologies and glomerulopathies (Table 5). The shift from CAKUT towards unknown causes in advanced CKD was also evident when the whole 2015–2024 period was assessed (Figure 7). Moreover, this analysis showed the increasing share of acute kidney injury (AKI) (Figure 7).

Table 5. Etiology of chronic kidney disease (CKD) in the years 2015–2019 and 2020–2024 in relation to the severity of CKD.

	2015–2019	2020–2024
Mild CKD (eGFR ≥ 60 mL/min/1.73 m^2) [N]	30	24
CAKUT [N/%]	14/46	14/59
AKI [N/%]	3/10	2/8
Genetic [N/%]	2/7	¼
GN [N/%]	2/7	4/17
Neoplastic [N/%]	3/10	2/8
SD [N/%]	2/7	¼
Unknown [N/%]	4/13	0
Advanced CKD (eGFR < 60 mL/min/1.73 m^2) [N]	17	32
CAKUT [N/%]	8/46	13/41
AKI [N/%]	1/6	3/9
Genetic [N/%]	1/6	3/9
GN [N/%]	1/6	4/13
Neoplastic [N/%]	0	1/3
SD [N/%]	3/18	0
Unknown [N/%]	3/18	8/25

CAKUT—congenital anomalies of the kidney and urinary tract; AKI—acute kidney injury; GN—glomerulopathy; SD—systemic disease.

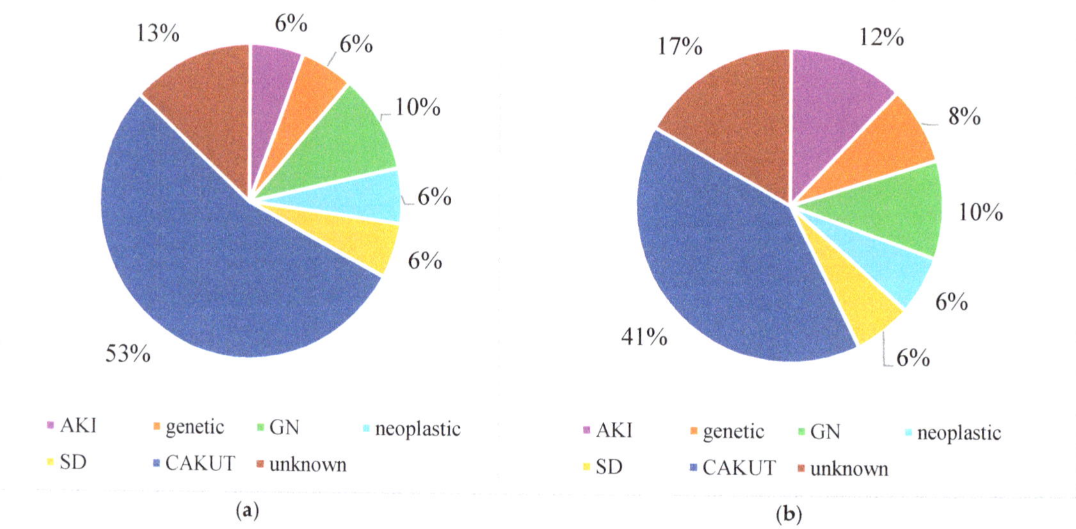

Figure 7. (**a**) Etiology in patients aged > 2 years with early-stage CKD (eGFR ≥ 60 mL/min/1.73 m^2) at diagnosis in 2015–2024 period; (**b**) Etiology in patients aged > 2 years with advanced CKD (eGFR < 60 mL/min/1.73 m^2) at diagnosis in 2015–2024 period; CKD—chronic kidney disease; AKI—acute kidney injury; GN—glomerulopathies; SD—systemic diseases; CAKUT—congenital anomalies of the kidney and urinary tract.

3.6. COVID-19 as a Causative Factor of CKD

In the analyzed cohort, there were only two patients who developed CKD in the course of COVID-19 as a probable infectious trigger. The first patient was admitted with a suspicion of AKI of an unknown origin and required dialysis. The routine PCR test was negative for COVID-19, but the child had high titers of IgG antibodies. No other infectious agent was identified, and no other probable reason for CKD was revealed. After 3 months, the patient's renal function improved (dialysis was ceased) but did not normalize, and CKD stage 2 was diagnosed.

Another patient was admitted to our department with a suspicion of AKI, anuria, and high parameters of uremic toxicity. There was no improvement after a few hemodialysis sessions, and symptoms of respiratory tract infection appeared instead. The patient turned out to be COVID-19-positive and was transferred to the ICU because of respiratory insufficiency. After steroid treatment, their general condition improved, but their renal function did not normalize nor improved, and the child remains dependent on dialysis.

4. Discussion

The COVID-19 pandemic created unprecedented challenges for healthcare systems worldwide, impacting not only the management of infectious diseases, but also impairing the diagnosis and care of chronic conditions, including CKD. The latter demands early detection, which is essential for slowing down the disease progression and delaying the incidence of complications. Thus, the pandemic may have further aggravated existing diagnostic difficulties, although no data confirming such a tendency exist.

Our data revealed delays in CKD diagnosis among children, confirmed by the significantly higher prevalence of children with CKD with eGFR < 60 mL/min/1.73 m^2 at diagnosis in the years 2020–2024 compared to the 2015–2019 period. In contrast, the prepandemic conditions provided more chances for early diagnosis of CKD, which was demonstrated by the domination of children with CKD stages 1–2 over those with advanced CKD.

CAKUT remained the major causative factor for CKD, irrespective of the age, sex, or analyzed time period. Its superiority was most evident in the youngest, accounting for 80% of cases in patients under 2 years of age. However, the dominance of CAKUT was still evident in older children. Not surprisingly, this fact translates into the long-term sequelae in the registries of adults with end-stage kidney disease, where CAKUT has become the fourth most common cause of incident kidney replacement therapy [8].

Along with the CKD progression, factors other than CAKUT increased their share under postpandemic conditions. The significant contribution of glomerulopathies was noticeable in mild CKD, whereas an alarming trend of a significant impact of unknown causes and AKI as reasons for CKD dominated when the late stages of CKD were taken into account. All of these could result from late referrals, but recent reviews shed new light on another probable trigger—kidney diseases caused by COVID-19 and able to progress to CKD.

Acute tubular necrosis was reported as the main scenario of renal involvement in the course of SARS-CoV2 infection among adults, while pediatric data confirmed AKI as the most frequent kidney complication of COVID-19 [9,10]. The possible explanation of further progression into CKD could be the concomitance of post-AKI damage and infection-triggered residual inflammation, although these theories have not been confirmed yet [11]. In the case of AKI-related CKD, the lack of regular follow-up in pandemic conditions could result in underdiagnosis or delayed diagnosis of AKI, followed by overlooking the progression into acute kidney disease (AKD) and faster progression to CKD. And yet, the issue is of paramount importance, irrespective of the underlying cause, once it is realized that up to 30% of pediatric AKI aggravates into AKD, which is then followed by CKD development in nearly 10% of cases [12].

A similar argumentation could be raised in the case of the increasing share of glomerulopathies. Collapsing focal segmental glomerulosclerosis was the main post-COVID de novo glomerulopathy among adults, whereas few reports described SARS-CoV2-associated cases of nephrotic syndrome in children [10,13]. No doubt, these data require careful verification and further analysis before an evident cause-and-effect correlation between the increased AKI/GN incidence among children with CKD and COVID-19-related kidney diseases can be proven.

Likewise, there is uncertainty about the probable connection between the increasing share of unknown CKD etiologies and COVID-19's influence on the faster progression of CKD. The adult data confirmed increased mortality and hospitalization rates among COVID-19 patients with pre-existing CKD, but no proof for faster CKD progression owing to infection exists [14]. Fortunately, the contribution of unknown causes among pediatric CKD patients is still lower than that in the adult population, exceeding 20% [8].

The interesting finding of our study was the dominance of male patients among all children with CKD, irrespective of the time period, age group, or etiological factors. Despite this discrepancy, there was no evidence for a higher incidence of CAKUT among boys with CKD. This finding requires prospective verification in the course of a larger study.

Taken together, these results suggest that pandemic conditions could add to the late referrals of CKD patients but had no major influence on the demographic data. The tendency towards increasing shares of AKI and glomerulopathies in the CKD etiology could be the consequence of COVID-19-related kidney pathologies, but no direct proof for a cause-and-effect relation has been presented so far. No doubt, this trend deserves further follow-up and prospective observations of children with CKD.

While waiting for hard data confirming the abovementioned hypotheses, another probable explanation for late pediatric CKD referrals that is worth considering is whether the healthcare system is deficient under unusual conditions.

According to a nationwide cross-sectional survey in Poland, almost 50% of surveyed adults experienced difficulties in the access to health services, where the main reported barriers included the prolonged waiting time, closure of medical facilities, or their restructuring into dedicated COVID-19 centers [15]. In order to ensure accessibility to healthcare, the Polish government established means of remote medical advice, such as e-visits. Nonetheless, the most affected medical consultations, which decreased in number, included the holiday and night care units in outpatient settings, home visits by physicians, as well as outpatient and home visits by nurses [16]. The public health areas that experienced the largest reduction in services were rehabilitation, screening tests, and periodic health checks, the latter being essential in preventive pediatrics. These limitations may have given way to underdiagnosis of chronic conditions that are characterized by an asymptomatic course until the advanced stages of the disease, such as CKD.

On the other hand, various data revealed a reluctance of self-reporting to healthcare units during the pandemic too. Observations among the healthcare providers in two Manchester hospitals estimated a 24.8% decrease in attendance at the emergency department between February and March 2020 [17]. Other data mentioned that nearly 32% out of 752 pediatricians who were surveyed by the British Paediatric Surveillance Unit and working in April 2020 at pediatric assessment units (PAUs) or emergency departments (EDs) witnessed a patient with a delayed presentation, mostly diabetes mellitus, but also sepsis and malignancy [18]. A further investigation among parents in Ireland documented that nearly 22% refused to attend medical units, although their children required healthcare [19].

No adequate Polish data exist, but pediatric nephrology units continued undisturbed service throughout the whole period of the pandemic and provided consultations for external COVID-19 pediatric patients suffering from nephrological complications. This constant availability of nephrological pediatric service is a probable explanation for the comparable numbers of patients with CKD who were admitted to our department in the 2015–2019 and 2020–2024 periods. And yet, the balance was shifted towards the late stages of CKD, which is pictured by the dramatic discrepancy between the median eGFR values in the years 2015–2019 vs. 2020–2024.

Whereas some publications focus only on the structural burden of the system during the pandemic, the child's accessibility to proper treatment depends also on the parental factor, resulting in a hesitancy of seeking medical advice under unusual conditions. Those parental concerns in the COVID-19 era could have a multifactorial background, such as misinterpretation of government restrictions of staying at home, fear of being infected during the visit at a medical facility, or an avoidant behavior, exaggerated by the stress of the global pandemic. Thus, the abovementioned reasons could also add to the delayed CKD diagnosis in pediatric patients during the pandemic. Hopefully, lessons taken from this pandemic experience will help avoid future similar obstacles.

On the other hand, the lesson taken from lockdown could be that of limiting COVID-19 spread among children, thus protecting them against SARS-CoV-2-driven CKD. Our two cases of post-COVID-19 CKD have shown severe, or even fulminant, clinical courses with irreversible renal damage shortly after infection.

We have to admit that our study has limitations. This is a single-center experience, so no national conclusions could be made. We did not have full access to the data concerning the availability of general pediatricians during the pandemic, so we can only speculate on the potential impact of restrictions in primary health services on late referrals to specialist care, resulting in a delayed diagnosis of CKD.

And yet, to the best of our knowledge, our study remains the first to investigate the impact of the COVID-19 pandemic on the CKD epidemiology in children. It confirmed the increased incidence of late referrals among children with CKD at the cost of less frequent diagnoses of children with early stages of the disease.

5. Conclusions

The process of diagnosing CKD was delayed in children under pandemic conditions. The disruptions caused by the COVID-19 pandemic, including reduced access to routine healthcare, delayed medical evaluations and placed strain on the healthcare system, which may have contributed to this trend. The increased incidence of late referrals could also result from parental behavioral patterns that were triggered by the unusual pandemic conditions. The direct translation of COVID-19-related renal damage into increased incidences of glomerulopathies, AKI, or unknown causes of CKD is yet to be established.

Therefore, further retrospective analyses of healthcare processes during COVID-19, as well as prospective observations of children with CKD who were diagnosed in the pandemic period, are needed to show the full spectrum of connections between different elements of the system and to create a preventive strategy for prospective crisis situations.

Author Contributions: Conceptualization, Ł.B., J.J., P.T., A.B. and K.M.; methodology, Ł.B. and K.M.; software, Ł.B. and J.J.; validation, Ł.B. and K.M.; formal analysis, Ł.B., J.J., P.T., A.B. and K.M.; investigation, Ł.B., J.J., P.T., A.B. and K.M.; resources, K.M.; data curation, Ł.B., J.J. and P.T.; writing—original draft preparation, Ł.B., P.T., A.B. and K.M.; writing—review and editing, K.M.; visualization, Ł.B.; supervision, K.M.; project administration, K.M.; funding acquisition, K.M. All authors have read and agreed to the published version of the manuscript.

Funding: This research received no external funding.

Institutional Review Board Statement: This study was conducted in accordance with the Declaration of Helsinki and its further amendments. The consent form for medical data access and scientific data analysis was distributed to all participants/guardians and signed on admittance to the Department of Pediatric Nephrology. Based on the University Hospital's ethical regulations for retrospective data analysis, there is a waiver from additional consent provided that no accessory biological material is taken/used and no additional investigations, exceeding routine diagnostic procedures performed according to the guidelines, are performed. Our data processing for the study fulfilled these criteria, so no additional decision was required.

Informed Consent Statement: Retrospective informed consent was obtained from all available subjects whose anonymized data were analyzed.

Data Availability Statement: The generated datasets are available from the corresponding author on reasonable request.

Conflicts of Interest: The authors declare no conflicts of interest.

References

1. Plumb, L.; Sinha, M.D.; Jones, T.; Redaniel, M.T.; Ridd, M.J.; Owen-Smith, A.; Caskey, F.J.; Ben-Shlomo, Y. Identifying children who develop severe chronic kidney disease using primary care records. *PLoS ONE* **2025**, *20*, e0314048. [CrossRef] [PubMed]
2. Harambat, J.; van Stralen, K.J.; Kim, J.J.; Tizard, E.J. Epidemiology of chronic kidney disease in children. *Pediatr. Nephrol.* **2012**, *27*, 363–373. [CrossRef] [PubMed]
3. Harambat, J.; Madden, I.; Hogan, J. Épidémiologie de la maladie rénale chronique chez l'enfant [Epidemiology of pediatric chronic kidney disease]. *Nephrol. Ther.* **2021**, *17*, 476–484. [CrossRef] [PubMed]
4. Zhao, W.-M.; Li, X.-L.; Shi, R.; Zhu, Y.; Wang, Z.-J.; Wang, X.-R.; Pan, H.-F.; Wang, D.-G. Global, regional and national burden of CKD in children and adolescents from 1990 to 2019. *Nephrol. Dial. Transplant.* **2024**, *39*, 1268–1278. [CrossRef]
5. Kidney Disease: Improving Global Outcomes (KDIGO) CKD Work Group. KDIGO 2024 Clinical Practice Guideline for the Evaluation and Management of Chronic Kidney Disease. *Kidney Int.* **2024**, *105*, S117–S314. [CrossRef] [PubMed]
6. Lentine, K.L.; Smith, J.M.; Miller, J.M.; Bradbrook, K.; Larkin, L.; Weiss, S.; Handarova, D.K.; Temple, K.; Israni, A.K.; Snyder, J.J. OPTN/SRTR 2021 Annual Data Report: Kidney. *Am. J. Transplant.* **2023**, *23* (Suppl. S1), S21–S120. [CrossRef]
7. Schwartz, G.J.; Munoz, A.; Schneider, M.F.; Mak, R.H.; Kaskel, F.; Warady, B.A.; Furth, S.L. New equations to estimate GFR in children with CKD. *J. Am. Soc. Nephrol.* **2009**, *20*, 629–637. [CrossRef] [PubMed]
8. Ortiz, A.; Kramer, A.; Ariceta, G.; Rodriguez Arevalo, O.L.; Gjerstad, A.C.; Santiuste, C.; Trujillo-Aleman, S.; Ferraro, P.M.; Methven, S.; Santamaría, R.; et al. Inherited kidney disease and CAKUT are common causes of kidney failure requiring kidney replacement therapy: An ERA Registry study. *Nephrol. Dial. Transplant.* **2024**, gfae240. [CrossRef]
9. Muthya, A.; Ekinci, E.I.; Lecamwasam, A. What is the spectrum of kidney pathology associated with COVID-19? *Intern. Med. J.* **2024**, *54*, 1935–1943. [CrossRef]
10. Baek, H.S.; Cho, M.H. Kidney complications associated with COVID-19 infection and vaccination in children and adolescents: A brief review. *Clin. Exp. Pediatr.* **2023**, *10*, 424–431. [CrossRef]
11. Nlandu, Y.M.; Tannor, E.K.; Bamikefa, A.T.; Makulo, J.-R.R. Kidney damage associated with COVID-19: From the acute to the chronic phase. *Ren. Fail.* **2024**, *46*, 2316885. [CrossRef]
12. Chisavu, F.; Gafencu, N.; Stroescu, R.; Chisavu, L.; Schiller, A. Outcomes of acute kidney injury continuum in children. *J. Nephrol.* **2024**, *37*, 2569–2578. [CrossRef] [PubMed]
13. Qi, L.; Deep, A.; Fox, J.; Yii, M.; Rahman, M.; Myint, M.; Myat, H.; Thet, Z. A scoping review on adult patients with de novo glomerular diseases following COVID-19 infection or vaccine. *Int. Urol. Nephrol.* **2025**, *57*, 447–462. [CrossRef]
14. Lin, Y.-C.; Lai, T.-S.; Lin, S.-L.; Chen, Y.-M.; Chu, T.-S.; Tu, Y.-K. Outcomes of coronavirus 2019 infection in patients with chronic kidney disease: A systematic review and meta-analysis. *Ther. Adv. Chronic Dis.* **2021**, *12*, 2040622321998860. [CrossRef]
15. Mularczyk-Tomczewska, P.; Zarnowski, A.; Gujski, M.; Jankowski, M.; Bojar, I.; Wdowiak, A.; Krakowiak, J. Barriers to accessing health services during the COVID-19 pandemic in Poland: A nationwide cross-sectional survey among 109,928 adults in Poland. *Front. Public Health* **2022**, *10*, 986996. [CrossRef]
16. Mrożek-Gąsiorowska, M.; Tambor, M. How COVID-19 has changed the utilization of different health care services in Poland. *BMC Health Serv. Res.* **2024**, *24*, 105. [CrossRef]
17. Isba, R.; Edge, R.; Jenner, R.; Broughton, E.; Francis, N.; Butler, J. Where have all the children gone? Decreases in paediatric emergency department attendances at the start of the COVID-19 pandemic of 2020. *Arch. Dis. Child.* **2020**, *105*, 704. [CrossRef] [PubMed]

18. Lynn, R.M.; Avis, J.L.; Lenton, S.; Amin-Chowdhury, Z.; Ladhani, S.N. Delayed access to care and late presentations in children during the COVID-19 pandemic: A snapshot survey of 4075 paediatricians in the UK and Ireland. *Arch. Dis. Child.* **2021**, *106*, e8. [CrossRef] [PubMed]
19. Nicholson, E.; McDonnell, T.; Conlon, C.; Barrett, M.; Cummins, F.; Hensey, C.; McAuliffe, E. Parental Hesitancy and Concerns around Accessing Paediatric Unscheduled Healthcare during COVID-19: A Cross-Sectional Survey. *Int. J. Environ. Res. Public Health* **2020**, *17*, 9264. [CrossRef]

Journal of
Clinical Medicine

MDPI

Article

Post-Dialysis Fatigue Is Not Associated with Serum Lactate Levels in Patients on Chronic Hemodialysis

Maurizio Bossola [1,2,*], Nunzia Ciferri [2,3], Ilaria Mariani [2,3], Tania Monteburini [4], Stefano Santarelli [4] and Enrico Di Stasio [2,5]

1 Servizio Emodialisi, Dipartimento di Scienze Mediche e Chirurgiche, Università Cattolica del Sacro Cuore, 00168 Roma, Italy

2 Policlinico Universitario Fondazione Agostino Gemelli IRCCS, 00168 Roma, Italy; nunziagiferri@gmail.com (N.C.); ilaria.mariani04@icatt.it (I.M.)

3 Divisione di Nefrologia, Servizio Emodialisi, Dipartimento di Scienze Mediche e Chirurgiche, Università Cattolica del Sacro Cuore, 00168 Roma, Italy

4 Dipartimento di Nefrologia, Ospedale "Carlo Urbani" Jesi, 60035 Jesi, Italy

5 Dipartimento di Scienze Biotecnologiche di Base, Cliniche Intensivologiche e Perioperatorie, Università Cattolica del Sacro Cuore, 00168 Roma, Italy

* Correspondence: maurizio.bossola@gmail.com

Abstract: Background/Objectives: To measure the peri-dialytic serum lactate, sodium, potassium, calcium, and pH and base excess in chronic hemodialysis patients with and without post-dialysis fatigue (PDF). **Methods**: Patients were asked "Do you feel fatigued after dialysis?" Each patient was invited to rate the intensity, duration, and frequency of PDF from one to five. The recovery time after the hemodialysis session (TIRD) was calculated, and inviting patients were to answer the following single open-ended question: "How long does it take you to recover from a dialysis session?" Pre- and post-dialysis arterial blood was sampled, and pH, bicarbonates, base excess, sodium, calcium, potassium, and lactate were measured. **Results:** One hundred fifty-eight patients were included in the study. One hundred seventeen patients declared to suffer from PDF and forty-one did not. Median [range] PDF frequency, intensity, duration, and TIRD were 5 (1–5), 4 (1–5), 3 (1–5), and 12 h (1–48), respectively. Seventy patients had a TIRD $\leq$ 12 h and forty-seven had a TIRD > 12 h. Median post-dialysis and post-dialysis/pre-dialysis difference serum lactate levels (mmol/L) did not differ between patients with and without PDF ($p = 0.111$ and $p = 0.395$, respectively). In addition, the distribution of patients according to post-dialysis serum lactate levels was similar in the presence or absence of PDF. The median post-dialysis and post-dialysis/pre-dialysis difference serum lactate concentrations did not differ significantly according to the score of the PDF intensity and PDF duration ($p = 0.928$ and 0.935, $p = 0.610$ and 0.548, respectively). Finally, we stratified patients into two groups according to the length of TIRD: $\leq$12 h and >12 h. The median post-dialysis serum lactate concentrations did not differ significantly between the two groups ($p = 0.862$) as well as the median post-dialysis/pre-dialysis difference ($p = 0.583$). Also, the distribution of patients according to post-dialysis serum lactate levels was similar in the two groups. **Conclusions:** PDF and TIRD are not associated with peri-dialytic changes in serum lactate in patients on chronic hemodialysis.

Keywords: hemodialysis; fatigue; post-dialysis fatigue; lactate; acidosis

https://doi.org/10.3390/jcm14082706

1. Introduction

Many patients, following a hemodialysis treatment, report to feel tired and the need for a rest or sleeping time. This condition, conventionally called post-dialysis fatigue (PDF), has been described as a feeling of being worn out, drained, or exhausted [1–3]. PDF is one of the most debilitating symptoms of hemodialysis patients, significantly impairing their quality of life and causing frustration and depression [1–3].

PDF is common, although prevalence estimates vary between studies from 20% to 86%, and differences in estimates are likely related to different inclusion criteria, ascertainment methods, or definitions of fatigue [1–3].

The causes and the pathogenesis of PDF are essentially unknown [1–4]. However, some mechanisms have been proposed, such as (1) the rapid decline in osmolarity occurring during dialysis as a result of the combined effect of a reduction in serum urea and sodium concentration (this leads to brain swelling and headache, restlessness, nausea, muscle cramps, and fatigue) [5,6]; (2) the release of cytokines such as interleukin-1, interleukin-6, and tumour necrosis factor-alpha [7–9]; and (3) the accumulation of metabolites and toxins in the muscle. In addition, the data point also to psychological factors contributing to PDF [1–4]. Referring to the third point, it has been suggested that intradialytic hypotension, one of the most common complications of hemodialysis, may contribute to muscle ischemia, accumulation of lactate in the muscle, high serum lactate levels, and consequent muscle fatigue and PDF [10–13]. These data are supported by the observation that higher levels of post-dialysis lactate are associated with PDF in patients on chronic hemodialysis and, in particular, that post-dialysis lactate levels in patients with severe PDF were significantly higher than that in patients with mild PDF [12]. It is hypothesised that microcirculatory dysfunction can cause regional tissue hypoxia and consequent hyperlactatemia [12]. Unfortunately, to the best of our knowledge, there is no evidence of other studies on this issue. The present study aims to measure the peri-dialytic serum lactate concentrations in end-stage renal disease (ESRD) patients on chronic hemodialysis and to define the possible correlation with PDF prevalence and characteristics as well with the length of the time of recovery after dialysis (TIRD) defined as the time taken to recover from a dialysis session.

2. Patients and Methods

All prevalent ESRD patients receiving chronic hemodialysis at our hospital in December 2024 were eligible for inclusion in the study. Exclusion criteria were as follows: dialysis duration <1 year, diagnosis of dementia based on DSM-IV criteria, presence of acute infectious disease, presence of active cancer, vascular access though a central venous catheter, heart failure, respiratory failure, haemorrhage, severe infections, alcohol abuse, shock, and liver disease [13]. The study was performed in adherence to the Declaration of Helsinki, and the protocol was approved by the local ethics committee (Prot ID 3169). Written informed consent was obtained from all participants before enrolment in the study. For each participant, the following parameters were recorded at the time of inclusion in the study: age, gender, underlying renal disease, weight, height, hemodialysis regimen, type and number of comorbid conditions, and the Charlson Comorbidity Index [14].

2.1. Identification and Grading of PDF

The assessment of PDF was conducted according to the studies of Sklar et al. [15]. Each patient was interviewed during one of the patient's regularly scheduled treatments. Patients were suffering from PDF if they spontaneously offered this complaint when asked the open-ended question: "Do you feel fatigued after dialysis?" Then, each patient was invited to rate the intensity, duration, and frequency of PDF from 1 to 5.

2.2. Other Measurements

The recovery time after the hemodialysis session (TIRD) was calculated according to Lindsay et al. [16]. Briefly, patients were invited to answer to the following single open-ended question: "How long does it take you to recover from a dialysis session?"

Functional ability was estimated using the Katz activities of daily living (ADLs), and the Lawton and Brody scale for instrumental activities of daily living (IADLs) [17,18]. These scales are most adopted for assessing functional independency for clinical and epidemiological purposes; disability in the ADLs was defined as need of assistance for performing two or more ADLs. The reason for not choosing a single-point decline is that impairment in two ADLs is less likely to capture physiological fluctuations in functional performance. Impairment in IADL function was identified by a score <7; this higher cut-off level is generally adopted to avoid a "floor effect". The ADL scale is based on seven levels of self-performance including dressing, eating, toilet use, bathing, mobility in bed, locomotion, and transfer. Similarly, the IADL scale is based on seven levels of self-performance including meal preparation, housework, managing finance, phone use, shopping, transportation, and managing medications. Finally, the Kt/V was calculated according to a standard formula and used as an index of adequacy of the hemodialysis treatment.

2.3. Hemodialysis

All patients received conventional 4 h bicarbonate hemodialysis three times a week. The blood flow ranged from 250 to 300 mL/min with a dialysis rate flow of 500 mL/min. All patients were treated with high-permeability membranes.

2.4. Laboratory Measurements

Blood samples were obtained from HD patients directly through the arteriovenous fistula before their scheduled HD session at the beginning of the week. Serum was separated within 30 min, and samples were kept frozen at −70 °C if not analysed immediately. Laboratory parameters were measured by routine methods at the Department of Diagnostic and Laboratory Medicine, Unity of Chemistry, Biochemistry and Clinical Molecular Biology. Pre- and post-dialysis arterial blood was sampled from the arterial blood line of the arteriovenous fistula, and the following parameters were tested: pH, actual bicarbonate, base excess, sodium, potassium, and lactate (arterial blood gas analysis).

2.5. Statistical Analyses

Statistical analysis was performed using the Statistical Package for Social Science (SPSS), release 15.0. Continuous variables were expressed as mean ± SD, categorical variables displayed as frequencies, and the appropriate parametric or non-parametric test was used to assess significance of the differences between groups. All data were first analysed for normality of distribution using the Kolmogorov–Smirnov test of normality. Correlations were calculated with the Spearman's rho correlation coefficient. After adjustment for multiple measures, a p-value < 0.01 was considered statistically significant. Correlation Matrix of Fatigue and hemogas analysis parameters were built, reporting Spearman's rho and significance values. The primary outcome was defined as the difference between pre- and post-dialysis serum lactate levels according to the presence of PDF or TIRD class (≤ or >12 h). Considering $\alpha = 0.05$, power = 80%, and the number of enrolled subjects, effect sizes of 0.51 and 0.53 were calculated for PDF presence and TIRD class, respectively; our observed effect sizes (0.1 units for both variables) are significantly lower, thus confirming the absence of association between lactate and PDF or TIRD. As shown in Table 1, no differences in baseline demographical, clinical, and laboratory characteristics between PDF presence and absence subgoups were detected, thus warranting no further confounding factor controls through the data analysis.

Table 1. Baseline demographical, clinical, and laboratory characteristics. Data are shown as mean ± standard deviation or median [95% CI for the median] for continuous variables. PDF: post-dialysis fatigue; CCI: Charlson Comorbidity Index; ADL: activity of daily living; IADL, instrumental activity of daily living.

	PDF Absent (n = 41)	PDF Present (n = 117)	p
Age (years)	66.2 ± 10.9	68.5 ± 11.2	0.256
Sex: male/female	31:10	73:44	0.179
Dialysis age, months	47.5 ± 45.6	54.5 ± 53.2	0.453
Primary cause of ESRD (n)			
hypertension	16	42	
glomerulonephritis	10	28	
diabetes	8	22	
interstitial nephritis	4	10	
polycystic kidney disease	2	9	
others/unknown	1	6	0.964
BMI	23.3 ± 3.3	23.8 ± 3.5	0.482
CCI	2 (0–6)	2 (0–7)	0.927
ADL	5 (0–5)	5 (0–6)	0.786
IADL	6 (0–8)	6 (0–7)	0.457
TIRD (hours)	2 (2 to 2)	12 (12 to 12)	<0.001
Weight gain (Kg)	2.7 ± 1.2	2.4 ± 1.3	0.254
Kt/Vurea	1.28 ± 0.4	1.32 ± 0.3	0.562
QB (mL/min)	268 ± 31	258 ± 34	0.146
Haemoglobin (g/dL)	10.8 ± 0.4	10.7 ± 0.6	0.377
Serum albumin (mg/dL)	3.63 ± 0.4	3.71 ± 0.5	0.412
Serum creatinine (mg/dL)	10.8 ± 2.5	11.3 ± 3.4	0.443
Dialysate sodium (mmol/L)	139 ± 1.2	139 ± 1.6	0.745
Dialysate temperature (°C)	36.4 ± 0.3	36.5 ± 0.1	0.195

3. Results

One hundred fifty-eight patients were included in the study. Their demographic, clinical, and laboratory characteristics are shown in Table 1. One hundred seventeen patients declared to suffer PDF (group A) and forty-one did not (group B). Median [95% CI] PDF frequency was four (five to five). Median [95% CI] PDF intensity was three (three to four). Median [95% CI] PDF duration was three (two to three). The median [95% CI] TIRD was 12 h (11.9 to 12). Seventy patients had a TIRD $\leq$ 12 h and forty-seven had one >12 h.

The pre-dialysis and post-dialysis serum pH and concentrations of bicarbonates, sodium, calcium, potassium, lactate, and base excess are shown in Table 2, either in patients with or without PDF. As expected, in both groups (A and B), a significant increase in pH, bicarbonates, calcium, sodium, and base excess and a significant decrease in potassium and lactate was observed between pre- and post-dialysis assessments.

Table 2. Laboratory variables and PDF. PDF: post-dialysis fatigue. Data are shown as median [95% CI].

	PRE-DIALYSIS			POST-DIALYSIS		
	PDF NO	PDF YES	p	PDF NO	PDF YES	p
pH	7.33 (7.31–7.46)	7.33 (7.31–7.34)	0.288	7.43 (7.70–7.46)	7.42 (7.41–7.44)	0.438
Bicarbonates (mmol/L)	18.1 (16.8–20.3)	19 (18.2–19.9)	0.512	23.3 (21.6–25.2)	24.2 (23.2–24.7)	0.604
Base excess (mmol/L)	−6.25 (−8.15–−4.63)	−5.9 (−6.9–−4.6)	0.670	0.5 (1.9–1.35)	0.5 (−0.4–1.25)	0.514
Sodium (mmol/L)	138 (137–139.2)	139 (137.6–140)	0.729	140.6 (140–141)	140 (139.9–141)	0.828
Potassium (mmol/L)	4.9 (4.6–5.2)	4.9 (4.7–5.3)	0.827	3.7 (3.6–3.8)	3.7 (3.6–3.8)	1.000
Lactate (mmol/L)	0.9 (0.8–1.2)	1.2 (1.1–1.4)	0.012	0.8 (0.2–1)	1.1 (0.9–1.2)	0.090

As shown in Table 3, the median [95% CI] post-dialysis serum lactate levels (mmol/L) and the median [95% CI] Δ post-dialysis/pre-dialysis serum lactate levels (mmol/L) did not differ between patients with and without PDF. In addition, the distribution of patients according to post-dialysis serum lactate levels was similar in the presence or absence of PDF (Table 4).

Table 3. Median [95% CI] post-dialysis serum lactate levels (mmol/L) and median [95% CI] Δ post-dialysis/pre-dialysis serum lactate levels (mmol/L) and PDF.

	PDF Absent (n = 41)	PDF Present (n = 117)	p
Post-dialysis serum lactate levels	0.8 (0.7–1.0)	1.1 (0.9–1.2)	0.090
Δ Post-dialysis/pre-dialysis serum lactate	−0.1 (−0.4–0.08)	−0.2 (−0.4–−0.1)	0.490

Table 4. Distribution of patients according to post-dialysis serum lactate levels and PDF.

Post-Dialysis Serum Lactate Levels	PDF Absent (n = 41)	PDF Present (n = 117)	p
0.5–2.0 mmol/L	41	110	0.191
2.1–4.0 mmol/L	0	7	
≥4.0 mmol/L	0	0	

The median [95% CI] post-dialysis serum lactate concentrations did not differ significantly according to the score of the PDF intensity and PDF duration (Table 5). In addition, the median [min–max] Δ post-dialysis/pre-dialysis serum lactate levels (mmol/L) were similar with regards to the PDF characteristics (Table 6).

Table 5. Median [min–max] post-dialysis serum lactate levels (mmol/L) and PDF characteristics.

	1	2	3	4	5	p
PDF intensity	1.1 (0.8–1.9)	1.3 (0.2–2.8)	1.1 (0–3)	1.1 (0.03–2.1)	0.9 (0.2–2.2)	0.516
PDF duration	1.4 (0.2–2.8)	0.8 (0.03–2.2)	1 (0.2–2)	0.8 (0–3)	0.9 (0.3–2.7)	0.057
PDF frequency	1.3 (0.4–2.8)	0.9 (0.2–2)	1.7 (0.6–2.1)	0.7 (0.3–1.5)	0.8 (0–3)	<0.001

Then, we stratified patients into two groups according to the length of TIRD: ≤12 h and >12 h. The median [95% CI] post-dialysis serum lactate concentrations did not differ significantly between the two groups as well as the median [min–max] Δ post-dialysis/pre-dialysis serum lactate levels (mmol/L) (Table 7). Also, the distribution of patients according to post-dialysis serum lactate levels was similar in the two groups (Table 8). As shown in

Figures 1 and 2, the correlations between TIRD and post-dialysis serum lactate levels and between TIRD and Δ post-dialysis/pre-dialysis serum lactate levels, respectively, were not statistically significant.

Table 6. Median [min–max] Δ post-dialysis/pre-dialysis serum lactate levels (mmol/L) and PDF characteristics.

	1	2	3	4	5	p
PDF intensity	0.1 (−0.1–0.3)	−0.1 (−1.5–0.6)	−0.3 (−1.8–1.2)	−0.2 (−2.2–0.9)	−0.4 (−1.9–1.1)	0.235
PDF duration	−0.05 (−1.8–0.8)	−0.3 (−2.2–1.1)	−0.1 (−1.5–0.6)	−0.3 (−1.8–1)	−0.3 (−1.8–1.2)	0.598
PDF frequency	−0.1 (−1.8–0.6)	−0.3 (−1.3–0.4)	−0.1 (−2.2–0.6)	−0.2 (−1.7–0.3)	−0.3 (−2–1.2)	0.986

Table 7. Median [95% CI] post-dialysis serum lactate levels (mmol/L) and median [95% CI] Δ post-dialysis/pre-dialysis serum lactate levels (mmol/L) and TIRD.

	TIRD ≤ 12 h (n = 70)	TIRD > 12 h (n = 47)	
Post-dialysis serum lactate levels	1.1 (0.8–1.2)	1.1 (0.7–1.3)	0.665
Δ Post-dialysis/pre-dialysis serum lactate	−0.2 (−0.3–0.1)	−0.3 (−0.4–0.03)	0.895

Table 8. Distribution of patients according to post-dialysis serum lactate levels and TIRD.

Post-Dialysis Serum Lactate Levels	TIRD ≤ 12 h (n = 70)	TIRD > 12 h (n = 47)	p
0.5–2.0 mmol/L	67	43	0.436
2.1–4.0 mmol/L	3	4	
≥4.0 mmol/L	0	0	

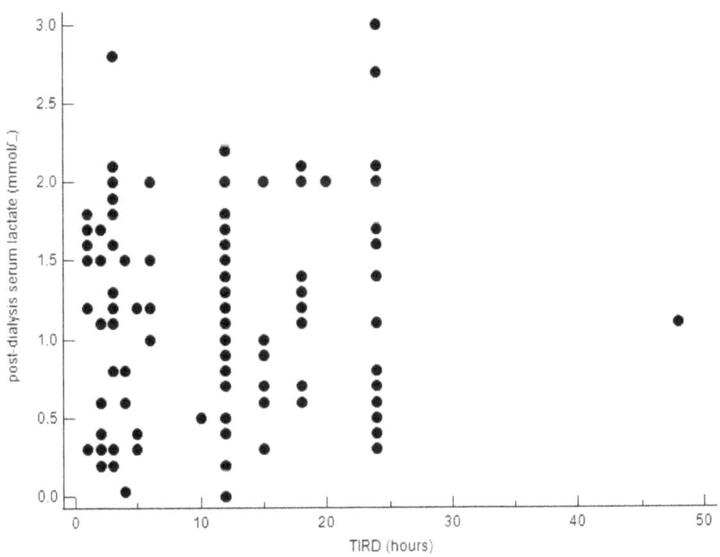

Figure 1. Correlation between TIRD and post-dialysis serum lactate levels. Correlation coefficient = 0.02504; $p = 0.790$.

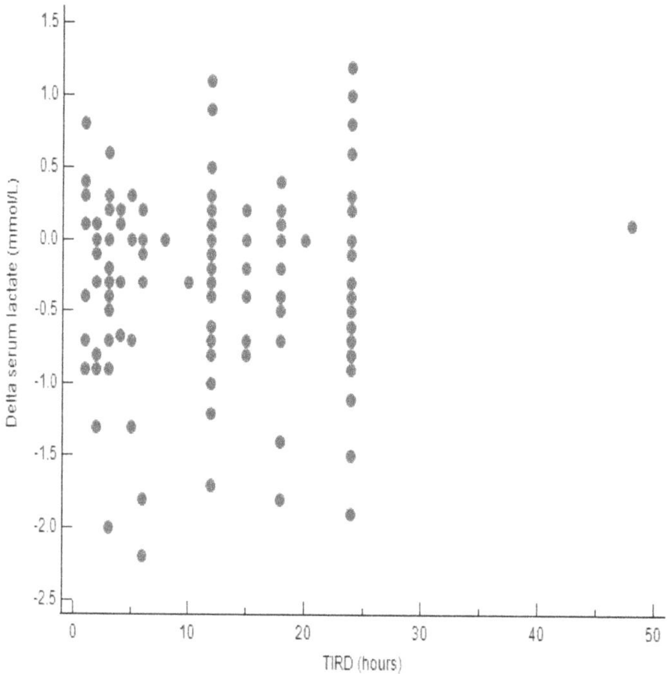

Figure 2. Correlation between TIRD and Δ post-dialysis/pre-dialysis serum lactate levels. Correlation coefficient = 0.017; $p = 0.843$.

Any significant associations between post-dialysis pH, serum base excess, and serum sodium and serum potassium levels with PDF, PDF characteristics, and TIRD were observed.

4. Discussion

The present study shows that the difference in peri-dialytic levels of serum lactate as well as the post-dialysis serum lactate levels are not associated with PDF frequency, PDF characteristics, and TIRD in patients on maintenance hemodialysis. These results are inconsistent with those of Zu et al., showing that mean post-dialysis serum lactate levels were significantly higher in patients with severe PDF than in those with no or mild PDF, and that higher post-dialysis lactate levels were associated with PDF [12]. With respect to the study of Zu et al., we did not stratify patients according to the severity of PDF (mild or severe). Alternatively, according to the study of Sklar et al. [3], we invited patients to grade the intensity, duration, and frequency of PDF on a scale from one to five. Interestingly, the median [95% CI] post-dialysis serum lactate concentrations did not differ significantly according to the score of the PDF intensity and PDF duration, and the the median [min–max] Δ post-dialysis/pre-dialysis serum lactate levels (mmol/L) were similar with regards to the PDF characteristics. This methodological difference in the assessment of PDF severity may, at least in part, explain the different results between our study and the study of Zu et al. [12].

Reference limits for serum lactate are reported as >2 mmol/l [19]. The present study demonstrates that the frequency of post-dialysis serum lactate >2 mmol/l and >4 mmol/L is similar in patients with and without PDF and in patients with TIRD length below and above the median value. Similarly, in the study of Zu et al., the frequency of post-dialysis serum lactate levels >2 mmol/l did not differ significantly among patients with no PDF, mild PDF, and severe PDF [12].

The results of the present study argue against the hypothesis that PDF may be the results of peripheral muscle metabolic alterations related to serum lactate levels. In fact, it has been suggested that intradialytic hypotension, one of the most common complications of hemodialysis, may contribute to skeletal muscle ischemia and consequent lactate accumulation, high serum lactate levels, muscle fatigue, and PDF [1–3,20,21]. In the present study, hypotensive event frequency did not differ significantly between patients with and without PDF, and this might explain, at least in part, the lack of association between PDF and serum lactate levels. Generally, accumulation of lactate in skeletal muscle and the consequent decrease in cellular pH have been considered to contribute to muscle fatigue [20–22]. However, the contemporary view is that lactate is no longer considered a metabolic waste product and cause of muscle fatigue but instead a myokine or exerkine with autocrine-, paracrine-, and endocrine-like functions [23–26].

In the present study, we also show that the association between the differences in peri-dialytic serum sodium concentrations with PDF, PDF characteristics, and TIRD were not statistically significant. Interestingly, some authors found that the post-dialysis serum sodium levels were significantly lower in patients with PDF than in patients without [12]. This discrepancy between our study and the study of Zu et al. [12] is difficult to explain and requires further study. Nevertheless, there is evidence that low dialysate sodium concentration leading to low post-dialysis serum sodium concentration is not associated with post-dialysis fatigue or general fatigue in patients on chronic hemodialysis [27,28].

Metabolic acidosis is commonly retained to be associated with fatigue in ESRD patients on chronic hemodialysis [29]. Indeed, there is lack of evidence to support this statement. Nevertheless, the observation in the present study of any significant association between the difference in peri-dialytic pH and serum base excess with PDF, PDF characteristics, and TIRD argues against this hypothesis. In addition, the increase in in intracellular muscle acidosis has been demonstrated not to be a central factor underlying the impaired contractile function in fatigued mammalian muscle [30].

We also found significant association between the difference in peri-dialytic serum potassium and PDF, PDF characteristics, and TIRD. It has been demonstrated, recently, that the membrane in patients on chronic hemodialysis is depolarised, mainly due to hyperkalemia, and it has been argued that this potassium-induced depolarisation resembles that in fatigued muscle [31]. In the present study, the pre-dialysis serum potassium levels (mmol/L) were 4.9 (4.6–5.2) and 4.9 (4.7–5.3) in patients with and without PDF, respectively, and this may possibly explain the lack of association with PDF and TIRD.

The present study has some limitations. First, being observational and crossover, no conclusion can be drawn about causality. Second, the single center of the study population can restrict generalisability. Third, the study relied on self-reported measures for PDF and TIRD. Nevertheless, numerous studies, in the past, have shown that these measures are accurate and reliable [3,4,6,8,15,16,28,30,32–35].

In conclusion, PDF is not associated with pre-dialysis, post-dialysis, and peri-dialytic changes in serum lactate in patients on chronic hemodialysis. Post-dialysis fatigue in chronic hemodialysis patients is a complex phenomenon and a multifactorial origin, with relevant roles of behavioural, social, and psychological factors [36]. Therefore, it is amenable to consider both, biochemical and psychosocial variables, when trying to unravel the aetiology of PDF in patients on chronic hemodialysis.

Author Contributions: Methodology, M.B. and I.M.; validation, I.M., T.M. and E.D.S.; formal analysis, M.B., N.C., I.M., T.M., S.S. and E.D.S.; investigation, M.B., N.C., I.M., S.S. and E.D.S.; resources, T.M.; data curation, M.B., N.C., I.M., S.S. and E.D.S.; writing—original draft, M.B., N.C., I.M., T.M., S.S. and E.D.S.; writing—review & editing, M.B., N.C., T.M., S.S. and E.D.S.; supervision, M.B. and T.M. All authors have read and agreed to the published version of the manuscript.

Funding: This research received no external funding.

Institutional Review Board Statement: The study was conducted in accordance with the Declaration of Helsinki and approved by the Ethics committee is of the Università cattolica del sacro cuore of Rome. The date of approval is 8 January 2011 (protocol number: P606/CE/2011).

Informed Consent Statement: Written informed consent was obtained from all participants.

Data Availability Statement: The data presented in this study are available on request from the corresponding author.

Conflicts of Interest: The authors declare no conflict of interest.

References

1. You, Q.; Bai, D.X.; Wu, C.X.; Chen, H.; Hou, C.M.; Gao, J. Prevalence and Risk Factors of Postdialysis Fatigue in Patients Under Maintenance Hemodialysis: A Systematic Review and Meta-Analysis. *Asian Nurs. Res. (Korean Soc. Nurs. Sci.)* **2022**, *16*, 292–298. [CrossRef] [PubMed]
2. Bossola, M.; Tazza, L. Postdialysis Fatigue: A Frequent and Debilitating Symptom. *Semin. Dial.* **2016**, *29*, 222–227. [CrossRef] [PubMed]
3. Sklar, A.H.; Riesenberg, L.A.; Silber, A.K.; Ahmed, W.; Ali, A. Postdialysis fatigue. *Am. J. Kidney Dis.* **1996**, *28*, 732–736. [CrossRef] [PubMed]
4. Bossola, M.; Marzetti, E.; Di Stasio, E.; Monteburini, T.; Cenerelli, S.; Mazzoli, K.; Parodi, E.; Sirolli, V.; Santarelli, S.; Ippoliti, F.; et al. Prevalence and associated variables of post-dialysis fatigue: Results of a prospective multicentre study. *Nephrology* **2018**, *23*, 552–558. [CrossRef]
5. Gordon, P.L.; Doyle, J.W.; Johansen, K.L. Postdialysis fatigue is associated with sedentary behavior. *Clin. Nephrol.* **2011**, *75*, 426–433.
6. Sklar, A.; Newman, N.; Scott, R.; Semenyuk, L.; Schultz, J.; Fiacco, V. Identification of factors responsible for postdialysis fatigue. *Am. J. Kidney Dis.* **1999**, *34*, 464–470. [CrossRef]
7. Dreisbach, A.W.; Hendrickson, T.; Beezhold, D.; Riesenberg, L.A.; Sklar, A.H. Elevated levels of tumor necrosis factor alpha in postdialysis fatigue. *Int. J. Artif. Organs* **1998**, *21*, 83–86. [CrossRef]
8. Brys, A.; Stasio, E.D.; Lenaert, B.; Picca, A.; Calvani, R.; Marzetti, E.; Gambaro, G.; Bossola, M. Peridialytic serum cytokine levels and their relationship with postdialysis fatigue and recovery in patients on chronic haemodialysis—A preliminary study. *Cytokine* **2020**, *135*, 155223. [CrossRef]
9. Bossola, M.; Di Stasio, E.; Giungi, S.; Rosa, F.; Tazza, L. Fatigue is associated with serum interleukin-6 levels and symptoms of depression in patients on chronic hemodialysis. *J. Pain. Symptom Manag.* **2015**, *49*, 578–585. [CrossRef]
10. Seong, E.Y.; Zheng, Y.; Winkelmayer, W.C.; Montez-Rath, M.E.; Chang, T.I. The Relationship between Intradialytic Hypotension and Hospitalized Mesenteric Ischemia: A Case-Control Study. *Clin. J. Am. Soc. Nephrol.* **2018**, *13*, 1517–1525. [CrossRef]
11. MacEwen, C.; Sutherland, S.; Daly, J.; Pugh, C.; Tarassenko, L. Relationship between Hypotension and Cerebral Ischemia during Hemodialysis. *J. Am. Soc. Nephrol.* **2017**, *28*, 2511–2520. [CrossRef] [PubMed]
12. Zu, Y.; Lu, X.; Yu, Q.; Yu, L.; Li, H.; Wang, S. Higher Postdialysis Lactic Acid Is Associated with Postdialysis Fatigue in Maintenance of Hemodialysis Patients. *Blood Purif.* **2020**, *49*, 535–541. [CrossRef] [PubMed]
13. Antinone, R.; Kress, T. Measuring serum lactate. *Nurs. Crit. Care* **2009**, *4*, 56. [CrossRef]
14. Di Iorio, B.; Cillo, N.; Cirillo, M.; De Santo, N.G. Charlson Comorbidity Index is a predictor of outcomes in incident hemodialysis patients and correlates with phase angle and hospitalization. *Int. J. Artif. Organs* **2004**, *27*, 330–336. [CrossRef]
15. Sklar, A.H.; Beezhold, D.H.; Newman, N.; Hendrickson, T.; Dreisbach, A.W. Postdialysis fatigue: Lack of effect of a biocompatible membrane. *Am. J. Kidney Dis.* **1998**, *31*, 1007–1010. [CrossRef]
16. Lindsay, R.M.; Heidenheim, P.A.; Nesrallah, G.; Garg, A.X.; Suri, R.; Daily Hemodialysis Study Group London Health Sciences Centre. Minutes to recovery after a hemodialysis session: A simple health-related quality of life question that is reliable, valid, and sensitive to change. *Clin. J. Am. Soc. Nephrol.* **2006**, *1*, 952–959. [CrossRef]
17. Katz, S.; Ford, A.B.; Moskowitz, R.W.; Jackson, B.A.; Jaffe, M.W. Studies of illness in the aged. The index of ADL: A standardized measure of biological and psychosocial function. *JAMA* **1963**, *185*, 914–919. [CrossRef]
18. Lawton, M.P.; Brody, E.M. Assessment of older people: Self-maintaining and Instrumental Activities of Daily Living. *Gerontology* **1969**, *9*, 179–186. [CrossRef]
19. Finsterer, J.; Milvay, E. Lactate stress testing in 155 patients with mitochondriopathy. *Can. J. Neurol. Sci.* **2002**, *29*, 49–53. [CrossRef]
20. Fitts, R.H. Cellular mechanisms of muscle fatigue. *Physiol. Rev.* **1994**, *74*, 49–94. [CrossRef]
21. Westerblad, H.; Lee, J.A.; Lännergren, J.; Allen, D.G. Cellular mechanisms of fatigue in skeletal muscle. *Am. J. Physiol.* **1991**, *261*, C195–C209. [CrossRef] [PubMed]

22. Finsterer, J. Biomarkers of peripheral muscle fatigue during exercise. *BMC Musculoskelet. Disord.* **2012**, *13*, 218. [CrossRef] [PubMed]
23. Brooks, G.A.; Osmond, A.D.; Arevalo, J.A.; Duong, J.J.; Curl, C.C.; Moreno-Santillan, D.D.; Leija, R.G. Lactate as a myokine and exerkine: Drivers and signals of physiology and metabolism. *J. Appl. Physiol.* **2023**, *134*, 529–548. [CrossRef] [PubMed]
24. Hall, M.M.; Rajasekaran, S.; Thomsen, T.W.; Peterson, A.R. Lactate: Friend or Foe. *PM R* **2016**, *8* (Suppl. S3), S8–S15.
25. Cairns, S.P. Lactic acid and exercise performance: Culprit or friend? *Sports Med.* **2006**, *36*, 279–291. [CrossRef]
26. Lee, S.; Choi, Y.; Jeong, E.; Park, J.; Kim, J.; Tanaka, M.; Choi, J. Physiological significance of elevated levels of lactate by exercise training in the brain and body. *J. Biosci. Bioeng.* **2023**, *135*, 167–175. [CrossRef]
27. Dunlop, J.L.; Vandal, A.C.; Marshall, M.R. Low dialysate sodium levels for chronic haemodialysis. *Cochrane Database Syst. Rev.* **2019**, *1*, CD011204. [CrossRef]
28. Bossola, M.; Di Stasio, E.; Monteburini, T.; Parodi, E.; Ippoliti, F.; Bonomini, M.; Santarelli, S.; Eugenio Nebiolo, P.; Sirolli, V.; Cenerelli, S. Intensity, Duration, and Frequency of Post-Dialysis Fatigue in Patients on Chronic Haemodialysis. *J. Ren. Care.* **2020**, *46*, 115–123. [CrossRef]
29. Kovacic, V.; Roguljic, L.; Kovacic, V. Metabolic acidosis of chronically hemodialyzed patients. *Am. J. Nephrol.* **2003**, *23*, 158–164. [CrossRef]
30. Westerblad, H. Acidosis is not a significant cause of skeletal muscle fatigue. *Med. Sci. Sports Exerc.* **2016**, *48*, 2339–2342. [CrossRef]
31. Larsen, L.H.; Z'Graggen, W.J.; Bostock, H.; Tan, S.V.; Buus, N.H.; Tankisi, H. The role of potassium in muscle membrane dysfunction in end-stage renal disease. *Clin. Neurophysiol.* **2021**, *132*, 3125–3135. [CrossRef] [PubMed]
32. Bossola, M.; Di Giovanni, M.; Mariani, I.; Di Stasio, E.; Angioletti, L.; Balconi, M. Post-Dialysis Fatigue Is Not Associated with Perceived Stress in Patients on Hemodialysis. *Hemodial. Int.* **2025**, *29*, 214–221. [CrossRef] [PubMed]
33. Bossola, M.; Monteburini, T.; Parodi, E.; Santarelli, S.; Sirolli, V.; Cenerelli, S.; Bonomini, M.; de Ninno, G.; di Stasio, E. Post-dialysis fatigue: Comparison of bicarbonate hemodialysis and online hemodiafiltration. *Hemodial. Int.* **2023**, *27*, 55–61. [CrossRef] [PubMed]
34. Bossola, M.; Picca, A.; Marzetti, E.; Pepe, G.; Antocicco, M.; Di Stasio, E. Post-dialysis fatigue and serum S100B protein in patients on chronic hemodialysis. A pilot study. *Ther. Apher. Dial.* **2023**, *27*, 471–479. [CrossRef]
35. Bossola, M.; Picca, A.; Monteburini, T.; Parodi, E.; Santarelli, S.; Cenerelli, S.; Sirolli, V.; Bonomini, M.; Di Stasio, E. Post-dialysis fatigue and survival in patients on chronic hemodialysis. *J. Nephrol.* **2021**, *34*, 2163–2165. [CrossRef]
36. Bossola, M.; Hedayati, S.S.; Brys, A.D.H.; Gregg, L.P. Fatigue in Patients Receiving Maintenance Hemodialysis: A Review. *Am. J. Kidney Dis.* **2023**, *82*, 464–480. [CrossRef]

Journal of
Clinical Medicine

MDPI

Article

Ten-Year Trend in the Potentially Inappropriate Prescribing of Renally-Dependent Medicines in Australian General Practice Patients with Dementia

Saad Alhumaid *, Woldesellassie M. Bezabhe, Mackenzie Williams and Gregory M. Peterson

School of Pharmacy and Pharmacology, University of Tasmania, Hobart 7006, Australia; woldesellassie.bezabhe@utas.edu.au (W.M.B.); mackenzie.williams@utas.edu.au (M.W.); g.peterson@utas.edu.au (G.M.P.)
* Correspondence: saad.alhumaid@utas.edu.au; Tel.: +61-362262190

Abstract: Background: There is limited published evidence on the prevalence of potentially inappropriate prescribing of medicines in relation to kidney function in older Australians, particularly those with dementia. **Objectives:** To examine the prevalence, temporal trends and factors associated with potentially inappropriate prescribing of renally-dependent medicines in patients with dementia, using Australian general practice data. **Methods:** This comparative study was reported in accordance with the STROBE guidelines for cohort studies. Retrospective analyses of the National Prescribing Service (NPS) MedicineInsight dataset were performed to determine the proportion of patients aged $\geq$ 65 years with a recorded diagnosis of dementia, along with matched controls, who had potentially inappropriate prescribing based on their estimated glomerular filtration rate (eGFR) during the study period (2011–2020). Each patient was included only once throughout the study. Potentially inappropriate prescribing was evaluated for 33 commonly used medicines, using the Cockcroft-Gault equation for estimated creatinine clearance or eGFR, in accordance with the guidelines from the Australian Medicines Handbook (AMH). Each patient's medicines were included if they were prescribed within 180 days after the most recent recorded lowest eGFR value for the patient. Medicines having prescribed doses exceeding those recommended for an individual's renal function were classified as 'inappropriate dosage', while those whose use was advised against were labelled 'contraindicated'. Both categories were regarded as inappropriate prescriptions. Descriptive statistics were used to summarise patient characteristics and medication use. Temporal trends were displayed in graphs, with statistical significance determined using the Cochran-Armitage test. Binary logistic regression models were used to examine the associations between sociodemographic and clinical factors and the prescribing of medicines inconsistent with AMH guidelines. **Results:** The unmatched cohorts included 33,101 patients, comprising 4092 with dementia and 29,009 without. Among them, 58.4% were female, and the overall median age was 8 years [interquartile range (IQR): 77–87]. After propensity score matching, there were 4041 patients with dementia and 8031 without dementia. Over the study period, potentially inappropriate prescribing increased slightly, but insignificantly, in both groups of patients; the prevalence of inappropriate use of at least one of the 33 drugs of interest rose from 6.5% (95% CI 4.5–9.1%) in 2011 to 8.9% (95% CI 6.0–12.7%; *p* for trend: 0.966) in 2020 in the dementia group, and 9.2% (95% CI 8.0–10.5%) to 11.1% (95% CI 10.3–12.0%; *p* for trend: 0.224) in the matched controls. Over the ten-year period, approximately 9.3% (377) of patients with dementia in the matched cohort received at least one potentially inappropriate prescription. Among these, 154 (40.8%) were for contraindicated medicines, and 223 (59.1%) were for inappropriate doses based on renal function. Among patients with dementia in the matched cohort, fenofibrate, nitrofurantoin, and moxonidine were the most frequently prescribed medicines at doses inconsistent with AMH guidelines. In the unmatched dementia cohort, potentially inappropriate prescribing was not significantly associated with demographic characteristics or most comorbidities; however, it occurred more frequently in patients with an eGFR below 30 mL/min/1.73 m^2 or those with concomitant diabetes. **Conclusions:** Positively, the prevalence of potentially inappropriate prescribing of renally-dependent medicines in primary care patients with dementia in Australia was similar to their matched controls. However, there was room for improvement in the prescribing of these drugs in both patients with and without dementia.

Keywords: dementia; potentially inappropriate prescribing; prevalence; kidney; dose

1. Introduction

Chronic kidney disease (CKD) is a common condition that frequently goes undiagnosed, especially among older adults [1]. This lack of recognition increases the risk of inappropriate medication use [2]. A key concern is the prescribing of renally-dependent medicines—those requiring dose adjustments or avoidance in cases of impaired kidney function—which remains a challenging issue in clinical practice [3]. Despite clinical guidelines, such medicines are often prescribed inappropriately to older patients with CKD [4]. In patients with renal impairment, inappropriate prescribing has been associated with significantly higher rates of adverse drug events, emergency department visits, prolonged hospitalisation, and, in severe cases, increased mortality [5–8].

Dementia is another condition that becomes increasingly prevalent with advancing age [9]. As the population ages, the number of individuals affected by dementia continues to rise, bringing serious challenges to clinical care and medication management [10]. Several factors contribute to the elevated potentially inappropriate medication risk in patients with dementia compared to those without, including cognitive impairment, poor medication adherence, polypharmacy, multiple comorbidities, and a higher likelihood of drug–drug interactions [11,12]. Communication barriers and reduced clinical monitoring may result in less individualized and suboptimal care [13,14]. Compared with non-dementia, those with dementia are also more likely to have additional chronic illnesses—such as hypertension and diabetes—further increasing their risk of polypharmacy [15]. Older adults with dementia are more likely to be prescribed five or more concurrent medicines and are at an increased risk of experiencing drug–drug interactions [16,17]. In advanced stages of dementia, clinicians may intentionally deprioritize renal dosing considerations in favour of a comfort-oriented approach, placing emphasis on symptom relief rather than long-term risk mitigation [18,19].

The coexistence of dementia and CKD presents a uniquely complex landscape for prescribing decisions [20]. Research consistently shows that individuals with dementia are more likely to receive potentially inappropriate medicines [11,12,21], a risk further heightened by impaired renal function [22]. Previous literature reviews have explored the prevalence and outcomes of potentially inappropriate prescribing in older adults with dementia, often employing screening tools such as the STOPP or Beers criteria [11,12,21]. However, these studies have not specifically considered CKD as a potential risk modifier for inappropriate prescribing within this population [11,12,21]. Our recent systematic review identified a notable gap in the literature surrounding the dosing appropriateness of renally-cleared medicines in older adults with dementia or cognitive impairment [23]. Based on the limited published data, we found that inappropriate drug dosing in such patients occurs frequently [23]. These considerations highlight the critical importance of careful medication management in older adults with co-existing dementia and renal impairment.

To date, rates of potentially inappropriate prescribing of renally-dependent medicines in patients with diabetes, hypertension, cardiovascular disease and atrial fibrillation have been well documented [24–27], but the frequency of potentially inappropriate prescribing and potential differences in older people with dementia, compared to those without dementia, have not been characterised. We aimed to examine the prevalence and temporal trends of potentially inappropriate prescribing based on kidney function, as well as the factors associated with potentially inappropriate prescribing, focusing on older Australians with dementia.

2. Methods

2.1. Design and Data Source

This comparative study was reported in accordance with the STROBE guidelines for cohort studies (Supplementary File S1) [28]. A retrospective analysis was undertaken using primary care data obtained from the National Prescribing Service (NPS) MedicineWise's dataset (MedicineInsight). The data spanned from 1 January 2011 to 31 December 2020. MedicineInsight contains anonymised patient demographics, clinical records, prescriptions, and pathology results from general practices nationwide across Australia. Demographic characteristics of the patients are largely representative of the broader Australian population in terms of age, gender and socioeconomic status [29]. Since the closure of NPS MedicineWise, stewardship of MedicineInsight has transitioned to the Australian Commission on Safety and Quality in Health Care. Further details on the dataset have been documented previously [30] and it has served as a data source for multiple published studies [1,24,31].

2.2. Study Population and Inclusion Criteria

For this study, we obtained records of patients aged $\geq$ 65 years, with and without a documented dementia diagnosis, from MedicineInsight. Patients with at least one recorded renal function test result, specifically the estimated glomerular filtration rate (eGFR), were selected for further analysis. Patients with at least three recorded general practice visits in the two years preceding the index date, defined as the date of the individual's most recently recorded lowest eGFR value during the study period (2011–2020), were initially included. Each patient was included only once throughout the study. Patients with dementia were required to have at least one year of data following their recorded dementia diagnosis, and those whose diagnosis date was not recorded or occurred after 31 December 2019 were excluded.

2.3. Study Outcomes, Study Covariates and Statistical Analysis

To identify potentially inappropriate prescribing, recommendations in the Australian Medicines Handbook (AMH) were applied according to the renal function of each patient [32]. We focused on a list of 33 drugs that are commonly prescribed in general practice and are recommended to be avoided or used with dosage adjustment in patients with renal impairment. The drug list was adapted from an earlier publication [25]. Only medicines that had clear dosage recommendations for renal impairment in the AMH were included (Supplementary Table S1). The included patients, both with and without dementia, had been prescribed at least one of the 33 drugs of interest during the study period. Each patient's medicines were included for analysis if prescribed within 180 days after the index date's eGFR test, with the latest prescription considered for the same medicine to allow more time for the prescriber to alter the therapy following renal function testing.

Medicines that were available in combination products were assessed for potentially inappropriate prescribing individually (e.g., metformin and sitagliptin). For each drug, prescriptions were marked as 'appropriate dosage' when the prescribed dose was in conformity with the adjustment specified in the AMH with respect to the patient's renal function [32]. Medicines were considered as having an 'inappropriate dosage' when the prescribed dose exceeded the maximum recommended for the patient's renal function. Medicines were considered as 'contraindicated' if the AMH recommended avoiding their use in renal impairment on the basis of the patient's individual renal function. Both 'inappropriate dosage' and 'contraindicated' prescriptions were treated as inappropriate prescriptions. It is important to note that the AMH recommendations use estimated creatinine clearance (CrCl), not eGFR, when providing guidance about prescribing for people with renal impairment. Our previous work showed that agreement between the eGFR and CrCl was excellent using the AMH, with 97% of the medicines rated as appropriately dosed by eGFR being also rated as appropriate using the Cockroft-Gault CrCl equation [25]. Prescriptions with no dosage or frequency recorded, or dosage documented as "take as directed" ("mdu") or "immediate", were coded as missing and excluded from the analysis.

Descriptive statistics were used to summarize sociodemographic and clinical characteristics of patients with and without dementia in both unmatched and matched cohorts, reported as medians with interquartile ranges (IQRs), percentages, or proportions. In the matched cohorts, we examined trends in the inappropriate use of at least one of the 33 drugs of interest among patients with dementia versus those without, spanning the period from 2011 to 2020. We first constructed a sample of patients without a documented diagnosis of dementia (controls) by matching them to dementia cases across the entire study period. Matching variables included age, sex, rurality, general practice location (by Australian state or territory location), socioeconomic status, index year, frequency of general practitioner (GP) visits in the preceding two years, and the presence of specific medical conditions. These comorbidities included heart failure, hypertension, stroke, atrial flutter, anxiety, arthritis, asthma, diabetes, deep vein thrombosis, depression, cancer, coronary artery disease, chronic liver disease, chronic obstructive pulmonary disease, atrial fibrillation, substance abuse, osteoporosis, chronic pain, and schizophrenia. Comorbid conditions were identified using algorithms that analysed both coded data and free-text entries within the 'encounter_reason', 'prescription_reason', and 'diagnosis_reason' fields [33]. The Index of Relative Socio-Economic Advantage and Disadvantage (IRSAD), developed by the Australian Bureau of Statistics (ABS), provides a summary measure of socioeconomic status across geographic areas based on census-derived variables such as income, education, employment, occupation, and housing. Higher IRSAD scores reflect more socioeconomically advantaged communities [34]. This index contributes to the ABS's broader Socio-Economic Indexes for Areas (SEIFA), which classify areas into quintiles ranging from 1 (most disadvantaged) to 5 (most advantaged) [34]. Geographic remoteness was assessed using the Accessibility/Remoteness Index of Australia (ARIA), categorised into five levels: major cities (ARIA 0–0.20), inner regional (0.21–2.40), outer regional (2.41–5.92), remote (5.93–10.53), and very remote (10.54–15) [35]. Due to the relatively small sample sizes in the outer regional, remote and very remote areas, these were grouped together into a single category. Thus, rurality was condensed into three categories: major cities, inner regional, and outer regional/remote/very remote. Additionally, the Australian Capital Territory was grouped with New South Wales, and the Northern Territory with South Australia, resulting in six regional categories: New South Wales/Australian Capital Territory, Victoria, Queensland, Western Australia, Tasmania, and South Australia/Northern Territory. Propensity score matching followed a 2:1 ratio (controls to cases) and was performed without replacement, in descending order of match quality [36,37]. Matching employed a calliper of 0.02

on the logit scale of the propensity score [38,39], and any absolute standardised difference equal to or exceeding 0.10 was considered indicative of a meaningful imbalance.

In the matched cohorts, the use of the 33 drugs of interest was quantified by drug class and active ingredient. The count and proportion of patients, both with and without dementia, who had inappropriate use of these drugs were summarised and stratified by eGFR categories ($\geq$30 mL/min/1.73 m^2 and <30 mL/min/1.73 m^2). For each year, we estimated the proportion of patients—with and without dementia—who were inappropriately prescribed at least one renally-dependent medicine. These estimates were accompanied by 95% confidence intervals (CIs), calculated using the exact binomial approach. Temporal trends were shown in graphs, and the Cochran-Armitage trend test was applied to evaluate statistical significance (accompanied by p-values from Pearson's chi-square analyses) [40]. To assess differences in proportions between individuals with dementia and their matched counterparts regarding inappropriate use of at least one of the 33 targeted medicines, a two-sample z-test was employed [41]. Additionally, a sensitivity analysis was performed to explore prescribing trends throughout the study period in both dementia and control groups without applying matching criteria.

We analysed sociodemographic and clinical characteristics of unmatched dementia patients using data from 2011 to 2020 to identify factors associated with the potentially inappropriate prescribing of at least one of the 33 drugs of interest. After checking multicollinearity, we performed a multivariate logistic regression. Peripheral vascular disease, initially part of the model, was excluded due to its multicollinearity with coronary heart disease. Moreover, variables such as general practice site (Australian state/territory location), number of GP visits in the past two years, Aboriginal and Torres Strait Islander (ATSI) status, number of renally-dependent drugs prescribed, and specific medical comorbidities (heart failure, atrial flutter, anxiety, arthritis, asthma, deep vein thrombosis, depression, coronary heart disease, chronic liver disease, substance abuse, osteoporosis, pain, and schizophrenia) were excluded from the model due to insignificance in univariate analyses. The dependent variable was the presence of inappropriate medication use, while the final independent variables included age, sex, index year, rurality, socioeconomic status, eGFR category ($\geq$30 mL/min/1.73 m^2 and <30 mL/min/1.73 m^2), and the presence of specific medical comorbidities (hypertension, stroke, diabetes, cancer, chronic obstructive pulmonary disease, and atrial fibrillation). A backwards selection procedure was implemented to determine the final regression model.

Data manipulation was carried out using SAS version 9.4 (SAS Institute Inc., Cary, NC, USA). Microsoft Excel 2019 (Microsoft Corp., Redmond, WA, USA) and IBM SPSS Statistics 29.0 (IBM Corp., Armonk, NY, USA) were employed for data cleaning and statistical analysis. Statistical significance was determined at a threshold of $p < 0.05$.

2.4. Ethical Considerations

This study received ethical approval from the Human Research Ethics Committee at the University of Tasmania (HREC Project ID 20006), along with approval from the MedicineInsight independent Data Governance Committee. As the data were anonymised, individual patient consent was not required.

3. Results

The unmatched cohorts included 33,101 patients, comprising 4092 with dementia and 29,009 without. Among them, 58.4% were female, and the overall median age was 82 years (IQR: 77–87). Patient inclusion is shown in Figure ??. The characteristics of patients in the dementia and non-dementia groups, both before and after propensity score matching, are detailed in Table 1. Through propensity score matching, we successfully paired 12,072 patients, including 4041 with dementia and 8031 without dementia.

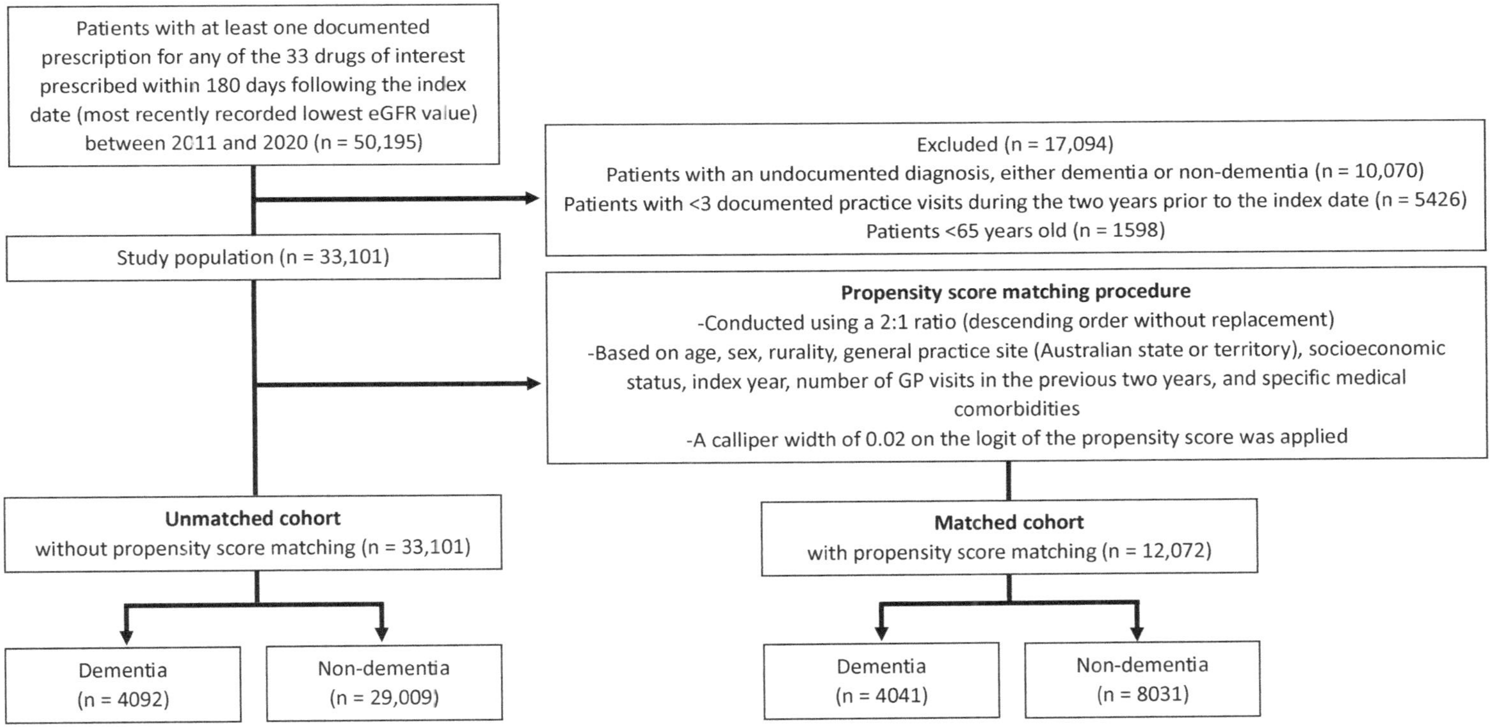

Figure 1. Flow chart of patient inclusion. GP, general practitioner; eGFR, estimated glomerular filtration.

Table 1. Baseline characteristics of dementia vs. non-dementia patients (2011–2020), pre- and post-propensity score matching.

Characteristics	Before Matching			Propensity-Score Matched		
	Dementia (n = 4092)	Non-Dementia (n = 29,009)	Standardized Differences *	Dementia (n = 4041)	Non-Dementia (n = 8031)	Standardized Differences *
Age (years), median (IQR)	81 (76–86)	82 (77–87)	0.167	81 (76–86)	81 (76–86)	0.005
Age group (years)			0.159			0.013
65–74	855 (20.9)	4555 (15.7)		840 (20.8)	1620 (20.2)	
75–84	1919 (46.9)	13,344 (46)		1895 (46.9)	3789 (47.2)	
≥85	1318 (32.2)	11,110 (38.3)		1306 (32.3)	2622 (32.6)	
Sex-female (%)	2355 (57.6)	16,982 (58.4)	0.016	2329 (57.6)	4641 (57.8)	0.003
Index year (%)			0.356			−0.014
2011–2012	913 (22.3)	4312 (14.9)		894 (22.1)	1906 (23.7)	
2013–2014	886 (21.7)	4755 (16.4)		874 (21.6)	1781 (22.2)	
2015–2016	825 (20.2)	4966 (17.1)		814 (20.1)	1486 (18.5)	
2017–2018	793 (19.4)	5974 (20.6)		786 (19.5)	1338 (16.7)	
2019–2020	675 (16.5)	9002 (31)		673 (16.7)	1520 (18.9)	
Aboriginal and Torres Strait Islander (%)			0.041			−0.017
Yes	31 (0.8)	191 (0.7)		31 (0.8)	48 (0.6)	
No	3284 (80.3)	23,807 (82.1)		3243 (80.3)	6418 (79.9)	
Unknown	777 (19)	5011 (17.3)		767 (19)	1565 (19.5)	
Rurality (%)			−0.091			−0.015
Outer regional, remote and very remote	2155 (52.7)	16,342 (56.3)		2150 (53.2)	4245 (52.9)	
Inner regional	1314 (32.1)	9170 (31.6)		1308 (32.4)	2743 (34.2)	
Major cities	591 (14.4)	3361 (11.6)		583 (14.4)	1043 (13)	
SEIFA quintiles (%)			0.041			−0.002
1 (least advantaged)	878 (21.5)	6214 (21.4)		872 (21.6)	1758 (21.9)	
2	995 (24.3)	6625 (22.8)		991 (24.5)	1998 (24.9)	
3	745 (18.2)	5359 (18.5)		739 (18.3)	1495 (18.6)	
4	690 (16.9)	4547 (15.7)		686 (17)	1147 (14.3)	
5 (most advantaged)	754 (18.4)	6141 (21.2)		753 (18.6)	1633 (20.3)	
General practice site (state location)			−0.055			−0.009
New South Wales/ Australian Capital Territory	1740 (42.5)	12,640 (43.6)		1713 (42.4)	3369 (41.9)	
Victoria	748 (18.3)	5956 (20.5)		742 (18.4)	1655 (20.6)	
Queensland	663 (16.2)	4486 (15.5)		656 (16.2)	1222 (15.2)	
Western Australia	332 (8.1)	1992 (6.9)		328 (8.1)	583 (7.3)	

Table 1. *Cont.*

Characteristics	Before Matching			Propensity-Score Matched		
	Dementia (n = 4092)	Non-Dementia (n = 29,009)	Standardized Differences *	Dementia (n = 4041)	Non-Dementia (n = 8031)	Standardized Differences *
South Australia/ Northern Territory	108 (2.6)	665 (2.3)		108 (2.7)	174 (2.2)	
Tasmania	501 (12.2)	3270 (11.3)		494 (12.2)	1028 (12.8)	
Number of visits to the GP in the preceding 2 years			0.019			0.007
3–5 GP visits	487 (11.9)	3043 (10.5)		479 (11.9)	874 (10.9)	
6–14 GP visits	1101 (26.9)	8235 (28.4)		1090 (27)	2284 (28.4)	
≥15 GP visits	2504 (61.2)	17,731 (61.1)		2472 (61.2)	4873 (60.7)	
Number of renally-dependent drugs prescribed (out of the 33 drugs of interest)			−0.009			−0.036
1 drug	2532 (61.9)	17,900 (61.7)		2501 (61.9)	5043 (62.8)	
2 drugs	1026 (25.1)	7570 (26.1)		1010 (25)	2068 (25.8)	
≥3 drugs	534 (13)	3539 (12.2)		530 (13.1)	920 (11.5)	
Comorbidities						
Heart failure	874 (21.4)	6959 (24)	0.063	861 (21.3)	1913 (23.8)	0.060
Hypertension	3072 (75.1)	22,290 (76.8)	0.041	3033 (75.1)	6039 (75.2)	0.003
Stroke	1055 (25.8)	5311 (18.3)	−0.181	1032 (25.5)	2030 (25.3)	−0.006
Atrial fibrillation	1268 (31)	9231 (31.8)	0.018	1253 (31)	2528 (31.5)	0.010
Atrial flutter	87 (2.1)	672 (2.3)	0.013	87 (2.2)	179 (2.2)	0.005
Anxiety	1161 (28.4)	5766 (19.9)	−0.199	1142 (28.3)	2242 (27.9)	−0.008
Arthritis	2874 (70.2)	20,483 (70.6)	0.008	2842 (70.3)	5631 (70.1)	−0.005
Asthma	711 (17.4)	5468 (18.8)	0.038	700 (17.3)	1378 (17.2)	−0.004
Diabetes	1370 (33.5)	9324 (32.1)	−0.028	1351 (33.4)	2655 (33.1)	−0.008
Deep vein thrombosis	83 (2)	657 (2.3)	0.016	81 (2)	178 (2.2)	0.015
Depression	1840 (45)	8103 (27.9)	−0.360	1802 (44.6)	3542 (44.1)	−0.010
Cancer	2064 (50.4)	14,171 (48.9)	−0.032	2031 (50.3)	3974 (49.5)	−0.015
Coronary heart disease	1336 (32.6)	9540 (32.9)	0.005	1315 (32.5)	2618 (32.6)	0.001
Chronic kidney disease	315 (7.7)	2384 (8.2)	0.019	312 (7.7)	580 (7.2)	−0.019
Chronic liver disease	35 (0.9)	233 (0.8)	−0.006	35 (0.9)	63 (0.8)	−0.009
Chronic obstructive pulmonary disease	758 (18.5)	5296 (18.3)	−0.007	745 (18.4)	1472 (18.3)	−0.003
Substance abuse	149 (3.6)	668 (2.3)	−0.079	144 (3.6)	278 (3.5)	−0.005
Osteoporosis	1499 (36.6)	10,775 (37.1)	0.010	1485 (36.7)	2928 (36.5)	−0.006
Pain	1972 (48.2)	13,779 (47.5)	−0.014	1948 (48.2)	3905 (48.6)	0.008

Table 1. *Cont.*

Characteristics	Before Matching			Propensity-Score Matched		
	Dementia (n = 4092)	Non-Dementia (n = 29,009)	Standardized Differences *	Dementia (n = 4041)	Non-Dementia (n = 8031)	Standardized Differences *
Schizophrenia	76 (1.9)	168 (0.6)	−0.121	65 (1.6)	93 (1.2)	−0.039
eGFR (mL/min/1.73 m^2), median (IQR)	53 (39–65)	51 (37–64)	−0.083	53 (39–65)	52 (38–65)	−0.035
eGFR category (mL/min/1.73 m^2)			−0.084			−0.061
≥30	3617 (88.4)	24,827 (85.6)		3571 (88.4)	6935 (86.4)	
<30	475 (11.6)	4182 (14.4)		470 (11.6)	1096 (13.6)	

* Absolute standardized differences are reported. Abbreviations: eGFR, estimated glomerular filtration rate; GP, general practitioner; IQR, interquartile range; SEIFA, socioeconomic indexes for areas.

Of the 33 drugs examined, rosuvastatin was the most commonly prescribed for both included patients with dementia (17.7%) and their matched controls (17.8%). This was followed by digoxin (11% and 11.9% for patients with dementia and matched controls, respectively), metformin (9.2% and 8.1%), and pregabalin (8.6% and 11%) (Table 2). The key changes in potentially inappropriate prescribing of the 33 drugs over time are shown in Figure 2 and Supplementary Figures S1 and S2. It slightly increased, but insignificantly, in both groups, from 6.5% (95% CI: 4.5–9.1%) in 2011 to 8.9% (95% CI: 6.0–12.7%) in 2020 (p-value for trend: 0.966) in the dementia group, and 9.2% (95% CI: 8.0–10.5%) in 2011 to 11.1% (95% CI: 10.3–12.0%) in 2020 (p-value for trend: 0.224) in the matched controls (Figure 2). The trend in potentially inappropriate prescribing calculated using unmatched dementia and control groups (sensitivity analysis) was similar to that obtained from the matched groups (Supplementary Figure S1).

Table 2. Renally-dependent medicines with potentially inappropriate prescribing in patients with dementia and their matched controls from 2011–2020.

Medicines ¶	Patients Prescribed N (%)		Patients with Inappropriate Use of Drug N (%)		Medicines ¶	Patients Prescribed N (%)		Patients with Inappropriate Use of Drug N (%)	
	Dementia	Control	Dementia	Control		Dementia	Control	Dementia	Control
Antidiabetic Medicines					**Psychotropic Medicines**				
Sitagliptin	8 (0.2)	30 (0.4)	<5	8 (26.7)	Paroxetine	70 (1.7)	156 (1.9)	<5	-
Alogliptin	-	<5	-	<5	Duloxetine	88 (2.2)	175 (2.2)	5 (5.7)	12 (6.8)
Saxagliptin	<5	<5	-	-	Risperidone	112 (2.8)	58 (0.7)	-	<5
Vildagliptin	<5	<5	<5	<5	**Anti-dementia medicines**				
Metformin	374 (9.2)	654 (8.1)	100 (26.7)	178 (27.2)	Memantine	35 (0.9)	20 (0.2)	-	<5
Antihypertensive medicines					Galantamine	29 (0.7)	47 (0.6)	-	-
Olmesartan	70 (1.7)	151 (1.9)	6 (8.6)	12 (7.9)	**Antihistamines**				
Valsartan	52 (1.3)	124 (1.5)	7 (13.5)	14 (11.3)	Famotidine	13 (0.3)	32 (0.4)	<5	13 (40.6)
Spironolactone	121 (3)	388 (4.8)	27 (22.3)	126 (32.5)	Nizatidine	36 (0.9)	72 (0.9)	10 (27.8)	35 (48.6)
Moxonidine	47 (1.2)	136 (1.7)	15 (31.9)	40 (29.4)	**Anticoagulant medicines**				
Antibiotics					Dabigatran	55 (1.4)	103 (1.3)	<5	11 (10.7)
Nitrofurantoin	64 (1.6)	108 (1.3)	40 (62.5)	72 (66.7)	Apixaban	197 (4.9)	371 (4.6)	8 (4.1)	29 (7.8)

Table 2. *Cont.*

Medicines ¶	Patients Prescribed N (%)		Patients with Inappropriate Use of Drug N (%)		Medicines ¶	Patients Prescribed N (%)		Patients with Inappropriate Use of Drug N (%)	
	Dementia	Control	Dementia	Control		Dementia	Control	Dementia	Control
Lipid lowering medicines					Rivaroxaban	180 (4.4)	330 (4.1)	44 (24.4)	77 (23.3)
Fenofibrate	49 (1.2)	105 (1.3)	33 (67.3)	67 (63.8)	**Neurological medicines**				
Gemfibrozil	7 (0.2)	30 (0.4)	<5	7 (23.3)	Pregabalin	346 (8.6)	886 (11)	<5	37 (4.2)
Rosuvastatin	714 (17.7)	1432 (17.8)	31 (4.3)	63 (4.4)	**Antiarrhythmics**				
Analgesic, antipyretic and anti-inflammatory medicines					Digoxin	443 (11)	954 (11.9)	<5	6 (0.6)
Diclofenac	71 (1.7)	157 (1.9)	<5	5 (3.2)					
Ibuprofen	55 (1.4)	94 (1.2)	<5	<5					
Indomethacin	30 (0.7)	39 (0.5)	<5	<5					
Mefenamic acid	-	<5	-	-					
Naproxen	41 (1)	102 (1.3)	<5	9 (8.8)					
Meloxicam	228 (5.6)	601 (7.5)	11 (4.8)	31 (5.1)					
Celecoxib	190 (4.7)	412 (5.1)	12 (6.3)	23 (5.6)					
Etoricoxib	<5	-	-	-					

¶ Combination medicines were assessed for potentially inappropriate prescribing separately. Note: cell counts less than 5 suppressed.

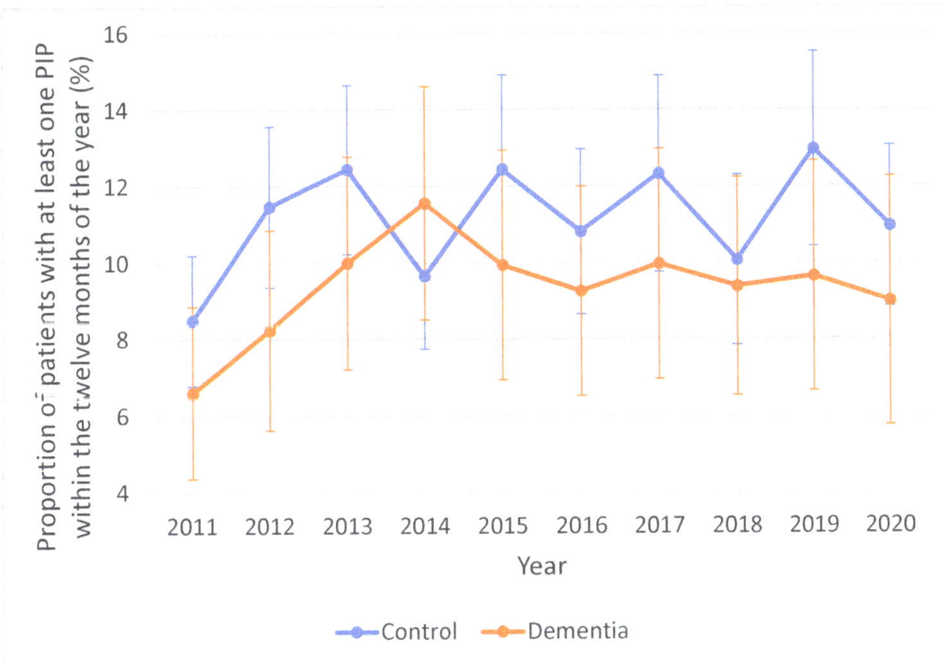

Figure 2. Trends in potentially inappropriate prescribing of 33 renally-dependent drugs in primary care patients with dementia and their matched controls. Error bars indicate 95% confidence intervals. PIP, potentially inappropriate prescription.

Across all study years, the prevalence of potentially inappropriate prescribing in the dementia group was slightly lower than that in the matched controls, except in 2014.

However, the differences were not statistically significant. Over the ten-year period, 377 patients with dementia (9.3%) received prescriptions for potentially inappropriate dosages, compared to 885 patients (11%) in the matched control group. Among the 377 patients with dementia, 154 (40.8%) received contraindicated medicines, and 223 (59.1%) were prescribed doses inappropriate for their kidney function. In comparison, 404 patients (45.6%) in the matched control group received contraindicated medicines, and 481 patients (54.4%) were given inappropriate doses based on kidney function. Among patients with dementia in the matched cohort, fenofibrate (33/49, 67%), nitrofurantoin (40/64, 62%), and moxonidine (15/47, 31%) had the highest proportions of doses that were inconsistent with AMH guidelines for renal impairment. In the matched control group, the highest proportions of such inconsistencies were noted for fenofibrate (67/105, 63.8%), nitrofurantoin (72/108, 66%), nizatidine (35/72, 48%), and famotidine (13/32, 40%) (Table 2). Across both matched cohorts, patients with or without dementia who had more advanced CKD (eGFR <30 mL/min/1.73 m^2) showed higher rates of potentially inappropriate prescribing compared to those in earlier CKD stages (eGFR ≥30 mL/min/1.73 m^2). Among patients with dementia and advanced CKD, the drug classes most frequently prescribed at doses inconsistent with AMH guidelines included aldosterone antagonists (spironolactone), alpha-2/imidazoline receptor agonists (moxonidine), antibiotics (nitrofurantoin), and fibrates—all of which showed 100% inappropriateness based on renal function. Similarly, in the matched control group with advanced CKD, these drug classes, along with H_2 antagonists, also showed 100% inconsistency with AMH guidelines (Supplementary Table S2). Sub-analyses based on eGFR severity (≥30 mL/min/1.73 m^2 and <30 mL/min/1.73 m^2) in the matched cohorts showed no statistically significant differences in the rates of potentially inappropriate prescribing between patients with and without dementia (Supplementary Figure S2).

From 2011 to 2020, sub-analyses across both matched cohorts were performed by age groups, gender, rurality, SEIFA quintiles, general practice site (Australian state/territory location), ATSI status, and frequency of GP visits in the preceding two years. These analyses revealed no statistically significant differences in the rates of potentially inappropriate prescribing between patients with and without dementia across the various sub-groups.

In the unmatched dementia cohort, variables potentially associated with at least one potentially inappropriate prescribing in patients with dementia from 2011–2020 were analysed through binary logistic regression analyses, and the results are shown in Table 3. Adjusted regression analysis revealed that patients with dementia were more likely to receive at least one inappropriate prescription if they belonged to the eGFR category of <30 mL/min/1.73 m^2, or if they had diabetes. Conversely, patients with atrial fibrillation showed a significantly lower rate of potentially inappropriate prescribing compared to those without this condition (Table 3).

Table 3. Odds ratio for factors associated with ≥1 inappropriate prescription in older patients with dementia (unmatched group) in Australian general practice from 2011–2020 (n = 381).

	N	At Least One Inappropriate Prescription, n (%)	Unadjusted		Adjusted §	
			OR (95% CI) ¶	*p* Value	OR (95% CI) ¶	*p* Value
Age						
<75	855	59 (6.9)	Ref		Ref	
≥75	3237	322 (9.9)	1.49 (1.12–1.99)	0.007	1.13 (0.82–1.56)	0.438
Gender						
Females	2355	210 (8.9)	Ref		Ref	
Males	1737	171 (9.8)	1.11 (0.90–1.38)	0.313	1.21 (0.95–1.54)	0.125

Table 3. *Cont.*

	N	At Least One Inappropriate Prescription, n (%)	Unadjusted		Adjusted §	
			OR (95% CI) ¶	*p* Value	OR (95% CI) ¶	*p* Value
Index year				<0.001		0.483
2011–2012	913	66 (7.2)	Ref		Ref	
2013–2014	886	96 (10.8)	1.56 (1.12–2.16)	0.008	1.34 (0.93–1.93)	0.122
2015–2016	825	80 (9.7)	1.38 (0.98–1.94)	0.065	1.14 (0.78–1.67)	0.510
2017–2018	793	76 (9.6)	1.36 (0.96–1.92)	0.080	1.08 (0.73–1.59)	0.693
2019–2020	675	63 (9.3)	1.32 (0.92–1.89)	0.130	1.32 (0.88–1.97)	0.173
Rurality				<0.001		0.661
Major cities	591	49 (8.3)	Ref		Ref	
Outer regional/remote/very remote	2155	197 (9.1)	1.11 (0.80–1.54)	0.521	1.14 (0.76–1.71)	0.520
Inner regional	1314	132 (10)	1.23 (0.88–1.74)	0.228	1.20 (0.81–1.76)	0.363
SEIFA quintiles				<0.001		0.310
1 (least advantaged)	878	78 (8.9)	1.15 (0.81–1.63)	0.442	0.81 (0.53–1.27)	0.369
2	995	100 (10.1)	1.32 (0.94–1.84)	0.110	1.11 (0.74–1.65)	0.624
3	745	75 (10.1)	1.32 (0.92–1.88)	0.129	1.20 (0.80–1.81)	0.371
4	690	66 (9.6)	1.25 (0.86–1.80)	0.241	1.14 (0.76–1.72)	0.524
5 (most advantaged)	754	59 (7.8)	Ref		Ref	
eGFR category (mL/min/1.73 m^2)						
≥30	3617	179 (4.9)	Ref		Ref	
<30	475	202 (42.5)	14.21 (11.22–18.00)	<0.001	15.13 (11.71–19.56)	**<0.001**
Comorbidities						
Hypertension	3072	321 (10.4)	1.87 (1.40–2.48)	<0.001	1.24 (0.91–1.70)	0.174
Stroke	1055	106 (10)	1.12 (0.89–1.42)	0.339	0.94 (0.71–1.23)	0.645
Diabetes	1370	200 (14.6)	2.40 (1.94–2.97)	<0.001	2.22 (1.74–2.83)	**<0.001**
Cancer	2064	200 (9.7)	1.09 (0.89–1.35)	0.400	0.94 (0.74–1.20)	0.624
Chronic obstructive pulmonary disease	758	67 (8.8)	0.93 (0.71–1.23)	0.620	0.80 (0.58–1.10)	0.167
Atrial fibrillation	1268	100 (7.9)	0.77 (0.61–0.98)	0.036	0.60 (0.46–0.79)	**<0.001**

¶ Odds ratio estimated using univariable and multivariable logistic regression with robust standard errors. § Adjusted for all variables. Abbreviations. eGFR, estimated glomerular filtration rate; GP, general practitioner; SEIFA, socioeconomic indexes for areas. Note: percentages do not total 100% owing to missing data.

4. Discussion

This study examined the prescribing trends of 33 renally-dependent medicines in the primary care setting for older adults with dementia. Notably, the prevalence of potentially inappropriate prescribing—defined as prescribing doses that exceed recommendations or involve contraindicated medicines based on renal function—did not differ significantly between patients with and without dementia. Approximately 9.3% of patients with dementia received at least one potentially inappropriate prescription, being inconsistent with AMH guidelines for renal impairment.

The drug classes most linked to potentially inappropriate prescribing were aldosterone antagonists (spironolactone), alpha-2/imidazoline receptor agonists (moxonidine), antibiotics (nitrofurantoin), and fibrates (fenofibrate). The medicines identified as potentially inappropriate for patients with dementia were largely consistent with previous studies on prescribing practices for individuals with renal impairment and dementia [22,42,43]. Antihypertensives and lipid-lowering agents are frequently prescribed for individuals with dementia [44], increasing the risk of polypharmacy and potentially inappropriate prescribing [21]. This is expected due to the common coexistence of hypertension and cardiovascular diseases with CKD [45]. Around 75% of patients were treated for hypertension, and 20% for cardiovascular conditions, including coronary heart disease, heart failure, and stroke. Many of these medicines are renally excreted, requiring frequent adjustments and heightening the risk of inappropriate prescribing [46,47]. Fenofibrate was the most frequently prescribed medicine at doses exceeding AMH guidelines (67% of cases). This aligns with findings from studies in France and Australia, which reported high rates of inappropriate fenofibrate prescribing in community-dwelling elderly individuals with impaired kidney function [26,48]. Fenofibrate is contraindicated for patients with an eGFR below 30 mL/min, yet it is sometimes prescribed for patients with an eGFR as low as 20 mL/min in clinical practice [49]. This may be due to patient-specific assessments, where cardiovascular benefits are deemed to outweigh the risks [50]. Severe hypertriglyceridemia and varying interpretations of guidelines among GPs also contribute to this discrepancy [49,51].

Of concern was the high proportion (62.5%) of nitrofurantoin prescriptions exceeding guideline-recommended doses in patients with dementia. A Canadian study reported that 100% of older adults with CKD Stages 4 and 5 in primary care received nitrofurantoin at inappropriate doses [52]. Increased resistance to sulfamethoxazole/trimethoprim and fluoroquinolones may explain the growing use of nitrofurantoin among the elderly [53]. However, decreased renal function, multiple comorbidities, and increased drug therapy in elderly patients necessitate careful consideration [54]. Reassuringly, the dosing of anti-dementia drugs, memantine and galantamine, was 100% appropriate in relation to renal function.

Prescriptions with potentially inappropriate prescribing showed no significant correlation with demographics or most comorbidities in patients with dementia, but were more frequent in those with an eGFR below 30 mL/min/1.73 m^2 or diabetes. Previous research on patients with advanced CKD has shown mixed results. While some studies indicate that enhanced monitoring and regular nephrology consultations reduced the incidence of potentially inappropriate prescribing [55,56], others have reported a higher frequency of prescribing-related issues [57–59]. Diabetes, a well-established risk factor for inappropriate prescribing in patients with CKD [26], frequently necessitates the use of medicines like biguanides (metformin) and DPP-4 inhibitors (sitagliptin, alogliptin and saxagliptin) [60]. These drugs often require dose adjustments in renal impairment [60]. Over 30% of our patients had diabetes, emphasising its influence on prescribed medicines, including frequent metformin use. Australian guidelines recommend annual assessments for renal impairment in individuals with diabetes [61], explaining more frequent eGFR monitoring by GPs in dementia patients with coexisting diabetes [62]. The lower rates of potentially inappropriate prescribing in patients with atrial fibrillation could be attributed to the structured guidelines and protocols for managing atrial fibrillation [63,64]. These guidelines emphasise the use of specific medicines and renally-adjusted doses [64,65]. GPs may also exercise greater caution when prescribing for patients with atrial fibrillation due to bleeding risks, resulting in more appropriate prescribing practices or even potentially under-dosing [66–68].

Studies suggest that a range of interventions—including computerised, manual, and educational approaches—can significantly reduce inappropriate prescribing in patients with CKD and mitigate associated adverse outcomes, with the most substantial benefits observed in pharmacist- or clinician-led initiatives [69]. These interventions should focus on renally-dependent medicines commonly prescribed to older adults with both dementia and renal impairment. Given the well-established association between potentially inappropriate prescribing of renally-dependent medicines and increased risks of adverse drug events, unplanned emergency department visits, prolonged hospitalisation, and mortality [5–8], healthcare professionals should prioritise addressing this problem in this vulnerable population.

Strengths and Limitations

To the best of our knowledge, no other study has looked specifically at trends of potentially inappropriate prescribing of renally-dependent medicines over time in primary care patients with dementia. Our study was based on a large, community-based nationally representative data source. It examined trends of potentially inappropriate prescribing over a 10-year period. Propensity score matching was used to adjust for patients' demographic and clinical characteristics. We also characterised whether prescriptions were consistent with guidelines utilising eGFR results which would have been available to the GP preceding the issuing of a prescription. We acknowledge several limitations in our study. Firstly, we did not investigate adverse clinical outcomes associated with potentially inappropriate prescribing. Secondly, the prescribing of seemingly inappropriate doses may sometimes be clinically justified in individual cases, where the benefits outweigh the associated risks or when no safer alternatives are available. Thirdly, the sample sizes for some of the individual drugs examined were relatively small. Lastly, the MedicineInsight dataset comprises unique patient records rather than distinct individuals, introducing a small possibility of duplicate entries for patients attending multiple practices.

5. Conclusions

In summary, the prevalence of potentially inappropriate prescribing based on renal function was not significantly different in patients with dementia compared to their matched controls. Approximately 9.3% of patients with dementia received at least one potentially inappropriate prescription that was inconsistent with the AMH guidelines for renal impairment. Such prescriptions were more common among patients with an eGFR below 30 mL/min/1.73 m^2 or those with diabetes.

Supplementary Materials: The following supporting information can be downloaded at: https://www.mdpi.com/article/10.3390/jcm14134734/s1, Table S1: List of medications which require dosage adjustment or avoidance with a reduction in renal function; Table S2: Renally-dependent medications by drug class with potentially inappropriate prescribing in patients with dementia and their matched controls with average eGFR ($\geq$30 mL/min/1.73 m^2, and <30 mL/min/1.73 m^2) from 2011–2020; Figure S1: Trends in potentially inappropriate prescribing of 33 renally-dependent drugs in primary care patients with dementia and their control groups without matching; Figure S2: Trends in potentially inappropriate prescribing of 33 renally-dependent drugs based on calculated eGFR category in primary care patients with dementia and their matched controls; File S1: STROBE Statement—Checklist of items that should be included in reports of cohort studies.

Author Contributions: W.M.B. and S.A. manipulated and prepared the data for analysis. S.A., W.M.B., M.W. and G.M.P. were involved in the manuscript's study design, concept, and revision. S.A. performed the data analysis and drafted the manuscript. All authors have read and agreed to the published version of the manuscript.

Funding: This research received no external funding.

Institutional Review Board Statement: Approvals were obtained from the University of Tasmania's Human Research Ethics Committee (protocol code 20006 and date of approval 10 April 2024), and the MedicineInsight independent Data Governance Committee approved the project.

Informed Consent Statement: All data utilized in this study were de-identified, and patient consent requirements were waived.

Data Availability Statement: The MedicineInsight data is now under the custodianship of the Australian Commission on Safety and Quality in Health Care (MedicineInsight@safetyandquality.gov.au).

Acknowledgments: We would like to thank general practices, general practitioners that contribute to MedicineInsight, and the patients who allow the use of de-identified information for MedicineInsight.

Conflicts of Interest: The authors declare no conflicts of interest.

Abbreviations

AMH, Australian Medicines Handbook; CKD, chronic kidney disease; CrCl, creatinine clearance; eGFR, estimated glomerular filtration rate; GP, general practitioner; NPS, National Prescribing Service; SEIFA, socioeconomic indexes for areas.

References

1. Jun, M.; Wick, J.; Neuen, B.L.; Kotwal, S.; Badve, S.V.; Woodward, M.; Chalmers, J.; Peiris, D.; Rodgers, A.; Nallaiah, K. The Prevalence of CKD in Australian Primary Care: Analysis of a National General Practice Dataset. *Kidney Int. Rep.* **2024**, *9*, 312–322. [CrossRef]
2. Aucella, F.; Corsonello, A.; Soraci, L.; Fabbietti, P.; Prencipe, M.A.; Gatta, G.; Lattanzio, F.; Cortese, L.; Pagnotta, M.R.; Antonelli Incalzi, R. A focus on CKD reporting and inappropriate prescribing among older patients discharged from geriatric and nephrology units throughout Italy: A nationwide multicenter retrospective cross-sectional study. *Front. Pharmacol.* **2022**, *13*, 996042. [CrossRef]
3. Hartmann, B.; Czock, D.; Keller, F. Drug therapy in patients with chronic renal failure. *Dtsch. Ärzteblatt Int.* **2010**, *107*, 647. [CrossRef]
4. Molnar, A.O.; Bota, S.; Jeyakumar, N.; McArthur, E.; Battistella, M.; Garg, A.X.; Sood, M.M.; Brimble, K.S. Potentially inappropriate prescribing in older adults with advanced chronic kidney disease. *PLoS ONE* **2020**, *15*, e0237868. [CrossRef]
5. Lohman, M.C.; Cotton, B.P.; Zagaria, A.B.; Bao, Y.; Greenberg, R.L.; Fortuna, K.L.; Bruce, M.L. Hospitalization risk and potentially inappropriate medications among Medicare home health nursing patients. *J. Gen. Intern. Med.* **2017**, *32*, 1301–1308. [CrossRef]
6. Clark, C.M.; Shaver, A.L.; Aurelio, L.A.; Feuerstein, S.; Wahler Jr, R.G.; Daly, C.J.; Jacobs, D.M. Potentially inappropriate medications are associated with increased healthcare utilization and costs. *J. Am. Geriatr. Soc.* **2020**, *68*, 2542–2550. [CrossRef]
7. Alyazeedi, A.; Fouad Algendy, A.; Sharabash, M.; Karawia, A. Prevalence, determinants and associated risk of potentially inappropriate prescribing for older adults in Qatar: A national retrospective study. *Clin. Interv. Aging* **2019**, *14*, 1889–1899. [CrossRef]
8. Su, S.; Gao, L.; Ma, W.; Wang, C.; Cui, X.; Liu, T.; Yan, S. Number-dependent association of potentially inappropriate medications with clinical outcomes and expenditures among community-dwelling older adults: A population-based cohort study. *Br. J. Clin. Pharmacol.* **2022**, *88*, 3378–3391. [CrossRef]
9. Tamura, M.K.; Yaffe, K. Dementia and cognitive impairment in ESRD: Diagnostic and therapeutic strategies. *Kidney Int.* **2011**, *79*, 14–22. [CrossRef]
10. Wang, C.; Song, P.; Niu, Y. The management of dementia worldwide: A review on policy practices, clinical guidelines, end-of-life care, and challenge along with aging population. *Biosci. Trends* **2022**, *16*, 119–129. [CrossRef]
11. Qin, Q.N.X.; Ming, L.C.; Abd Wahab, M.S.; Tan, C.S.; Yuda, A.; Hermansyah, A. Drug-related problems among older people with dementia: A systematic review. *Res. Soc. Adm. Pharm.* **2023**, *19*, 873–881. [CrossRef]
12. Zhao, M.; Chen, Z.; Xu, T.; Fan, P.; Tian, F. Global prevalence of polypharmacy and potentially inappropriate medication in older patients with dementia: A systematic review and meta-analysis. *Front. Pharmacol.* **2023**, *14*, 1221069. [CrossRef] [PubMed]
13. Bergman, H.; Borson, S.; Jessen, F.; Krolak-Salmon, P.; Pirani, A.; Rasmussen, J.; Rodrigo, J.; Taddeo, D. Dementia and comorbidities in primary care: A scoping review. *BMC Prim. Care* **2023**, *24*, 277. [CrossRef] [PubMed]
14. Hamiduzzaman, M.; Kuot, A.; Greenhill, J.; Strivens, E.; Isaac, V. Towards personalized care: Factors associated with the quality of life of residents with dementia in Australian rural aged care homes. *PLoS ONE* **2020**, *15*, e0233450. [CrossRef] [PubMed]
15. Clague, F.; Mercer, S.W.; McLean, G.; Reynish, E.; Guthrie, B. Comorbidity and polypharmacy in people with dementia: Insights from a large, population-based cross-sectional analysis of primary care data. *Age Ageing* **2017**, *46*, 33–39. [CrossRef]
16. Ruangritchankul, S.; Peel, N.M.; Hanjani, L.S.; Gray, L.C. Drug related problems in older adults living with dementia. *PLoS ONE* **2020**, *15*, e0236830. [CrossRef]
17. Banta, J.E. *Dementia: Morbidity and Medications*; Oxford University Press: Oxford, UK, 2017; pp. 4–5.
18. Mitchell, S.L.; Teno, J.M.; Kiely, D.K.; Shaffer, M.L.; Jones, R.N.; Prigerson, H.G.; Volicer, L.; Givens, J.L.; Hamel, M.B. The clinical course of advanced dementia. *N. Engl. J. Med.* **2009**, *361*, 1529–1538. [CrossRef]
19. Scott, J.; Owen-Smith, A.; Tonkin-Crine, S.; Rayner, H.; Roderick, P.; Okamoto, I.; Leydon, G.; Caskey, F.; Methven, S. Decision-making for people with dementia and advanced kidney disease: A secondary qualitative analysis of interviews from the Conservative Kidney Management Assessment of Practice Patterns Study. *BMJ Open* **2018**, *8*, e022385. [CrossRef]

20. Pépin, M.; Giannakou, K.; Levassort, H.; Farinha, A.; Bobot, M.; Lo Re, V.; Golenia, A.; Małyszko, J.; Mattace-Raso, F.; Klimkowcz-Mrowiec, A. Care pathways for patients with cognitive impairment and chronic kidney disease. *Nephrol. Dial. Transplant.* **2025**, *40*, ii28–ii36. [CrossRef]
21. Delgado, J.; Bowman, K.; Clare, L. Potentially inappropriate prescribing in dementia: A state-of-the-art review since 2007. *BMJ Open* **2020**, *10*, e029172. [CrossRef]
22. Sönnerstam, E.; Sjölander, M.; Gustafsson, M. Inappropriate prescription and renal function among older patients with cognitive impairment. *Drugs Aging* **2016**, *33*, 889–899. [CrossRef]
23. Alhumaid, S.; Bezabhe, W.M.; Williams, M.; Peterson, G.M. Prevalence and Risk Factors of Inappropriate Drug Dosing among Older Adults with Dementia or Cognitive Impairment and Renal Impairment: A Systematic Review. *J. Clin. Med.* **2024**, *13*, 5658. [CrossRef] [PubMed]
24. Bezabhe, W.M.; Bereznicki, L.R.; Radford, J.; Wimmer, B.C.; Salahudeen, M.S.; Peterson, G.M. Eight-year trends in direct-acting oral anticoagulant dosing, based on age and kidney function, in patients with atrial fibrillation. *J. Patient Saf.* **2022**, *18*, 337–341. [CrossRef]
25. Castelino, R.L.; Saunder, T.; Kitsos, A.; Peterson, G.M.; Jose, M.; Wimmer, B.; Khanam, M.; Bezabhe, W.; Stankovich, J.; Radford, J. Quality use of medicines in patients with chronic kidney disease. *BMC Nephrol.* **2020**, *21*, 216. [CrossRef] [PubMed]
26. Khanal, A.; Peterson, G.M.; Castelino, R.L.; Jose, M.D. Potentially inappropriate prescribing of renally cleared drugs in elderly patients in community and aged care settings. *Drugs Aging* **2015**, *32*, 391–400. [CrossRef]
27. Manski-Nankervis, J.-A.; Thuraisingam, S.; Sluggett, J.K.; Kilov, G.; Furler, J.; O'Neal, D.; Jenkins, A. Prescribing of diabetes medications to people with type 2 diabetes and chronic kidney disease: A national cross-sectional study. *BMC Fam. Pract.* **2019**, *20*, 29. [CrossRef] [PubMed]
28. Von Elm, E.; Altman, D.G.; Egger, M.; Pocock, S.J.; Gøtzsche, P.C.; Vandenbroucke, J.P. The Strengthening the Reporting of Observational Studies in Epidemiology (STROBE) statement: Guidelines for reporting observational studies. *Lancet* **2007**, *370*, 1453–1457. [CrossRef]
29. Busingye, D.M.R.; Mina, R.; Thistlethwaite, J.; Belcher, J.; Chidwick, K. *MedicineInsight Report: Validation of the MedicineInsight Database: Completeness, Generalisability and Plausibility*; NPS MedicineWise: Sydney, Australia, 2020. Available online: https://www.nps.org.au/assets/MedicineInsight-Validation-completeness-representativeness-plausibility_2020.pdf (accessed on 14 November 2024).
30. Busingye, D.; Gianacas, C.; Pollack, A.; Chidwick, K.; Merrifield, A.; Norman, S.; Mullin, B.; Hayhurst, R.; Blogg, S.; Havard, A. Data Resource Profile: MedicineInsight, an Australian national primary health care database. *Int. J. Epidemiol.* **2019**, *48*, 1741–1741h. [CrossRef]
31. Khanam, M.A.; Kitsos, A.; Stankovich, J.; Castelino, R.; Jose, M.; Peterson, G.M.; Wimmer, B.; Zaidi, T.R.; Radford, J. Association of continuity of care with blood pressure control in patients with chronic kidney disease and hypertension. *Aust. J. Gen. Pract.* **2019**, *48*, 300–306. [CrossRef]
32. *Australian Medicines Handbook 2024 (Online)*; Australian Medicines Handbook Pty Ltd.: Adelaide, Australia, 2024. Available online: https://amhonline.amh.net.au (accessed on 14 November 2024).
33. NPS MedicineWise. *MedicineInsight Databook*; NPS MedicineWise: Sydney, Australia, 2021. Available online: https://www.nps.org.au/assets/NPS/pdf/MedicineInsight-databook-4.0-December-2021.pdf (accessed on 14 November 2024).
34. Australian Bureau of Statistics. Socio-Economic Indexes for Areas (SEIFA). Available online: https://www.abs.gov.au/websitedbs/censushome.nsf/home/seifa (accessed on 14 November 2024).
35. Australian Bureau of Statistics. Australian Statistical Geography Standard (ASGS): Volume 5—Remoteness Structure, July 2016. Defining Remoteness Areas. Available online: https://www.abs.gov.au/ausstats/abs@.nsf/Latestproducts/1270.0.55.005Main%20Features15July%202016?opendocument&tabname=Summary&prodno=1270.0.55.005&issue=July%202016&num=&view= (accessed on 14 November 2024).
36. Iwagami, M.; Shinozaki, T. Introduction to matching in case-control and cohort studies. *Ann. Clin. Epidemiol.* **2022**, *4*, 33–40. [CrossRef]
37. Ripollone, J.E.; Huybrechts, K.F.; Rothman, K.J.; Ferguson, R.E.; Franklin, J.M. Implications of the propensity score matching paradox in pharmacoepidemiology. *Am. J. Epidemiol.* **2018**, *187*, 1951–1961. [CrossRef] [PubMed]
38. Friberg, L.; Andersson, T.; Rosenqvist, M. Less dementia and stroke in low-risk patients with atrial fibrillation taking oral anticoagulation. *Eur. Heart J.* **2019**, *40*, 2327–2335. [CrossRef]
39. Austin, P.C. Propensity-score matching in the cardiovascular surgery literature from 2004 to 2006: A systematic review and suggestions for improvement. *J. Thorac. Cardiovasc. Surg.* **2007**, *134*, 1128–1135.e3. [CrossRef] [PubMed]
40. Lachin, J.M. Power and sample size evaluation for the Cochran–Mantel–Haenszel mean score (Wilcoxon rank sum) test and the Cochran–Armitage test for trend. *Stat. Med.* **2011**, *30*, 3057–3066. [CrossRef]

41. Weisburd, D.; Britt, C.; Wilson, D.B.; Wooditch, A.; Weisburd, D.; Britt, C.; Wilson, D.B.; Wooditch, A. Comparing Means and Proportions in Two Samples to Test Hypotheses About Population Parameters. In *Basic Statistics in Criminology and Criminal Justice*; Springer: Cham, Switzerland, 2020; pp. 315–371.
42. Pfister, B.; Jonsson, J.; Gustafsson, M. Drug-related problems and medication reviews among old people with dementia. *BMC Pharmacol. Toxicol.* **2017**, *18*, 52. [CrossRef]
43. Delgado, J.; Jones, L.; Bradley, M.C.; Allan, L.M.; Ballard, C.; Clare, L.; Fortinsky, R.H.; Hughes, C.M.; Melzer, D. Potentially inappropriate prescribing in dementia, multi-morbidity and incidence of adverse health outcomes. *Age Ageing* **2021**, *50*, 457–464. [CrossRef]
44. Lau, E.C.Y.; Jeon, Y.H.; Hilmer, S.N.; Tan, E.C. Prescribing patterns in people living with dementia in the community: A cross-sectional study. *Australas. J. Ageing* **2025**, *44*, e13380. [CrossRef] [PubMed]
45. Hamrahian, S.M. Hypertension and cardiovascular disease in patients with chronic kidney disease. In *Approaches to Chronic Kidney Disease: A Guide for Primary Care Providers and Non-Nephrologists*; Springer: Cham, Switzerland, 2021; pp. 281–295.
46. Dincer, N.; Dagel, T.; Afsar, B.; Covic, A.; Ortiz, A.; Kanbay, M. The effect of chronic kidney disease on lipid metabolism. *Int. Urol. Nephrol.* **2019**, *51*, 265–277. [CrossRef]
47. Sinha, A.D.; Agarwal, R. Clinical pharmacology of antihypertensive therapy for the treatment of hypertension in CKD. *Clin. J. Am. Soc. Nephrol.* **2019**, *14*, 757–764. [CrossRef]
48. Breton, G.; Froissart, M.; Janus, N.; Launay-Vacher, V.; Berr, C.; Tzourio, C.; Helmer, C.; Stengel, B. Inappropriate drug use and mortality in community-dwelling elderly with impaired kidney function—The Three-City population-based study. *Nephrol. Dial. Transplant.* **2011**, *26*, 2852–2859. [CrossRef]
49. Therapeutic Guidelines Limited. *Therapeutic Guidelines: Cardiovascular. Lipid Modification. Version 21*; Therapeutic Guidelines Limited: North Melbourne, VIC, Australia, 2025. Available online: https://app-tg-org-au.ezproxy.utas.edu.au/viewTopic?etgAccess=true&guidelinePage=Cardiovascular&topicfile=cardiovascular-disease-risk-stratification&guidelinename=auto&sectionId=r_CVG_Lipid-modificationtopic_28#r_CVG_Lipid-modificationtopic_28 (accessed on 14 April 2025).
50. Wiggins, B.S.; Saseen, J.J.; Page, R.L.; Reed, B.N.; Sneed, K.; Kostis, J.B.; Lanfear, D.; Virani, S.; Morris, P.B. Recommendations for management of clinically significant drug-drug interactions with statins and select agents used in patients with cardiovascular disease: A scientific statement from the American Heart Association. *Circulation* **2016**, *134*, e468–e495. [CrossRef]
51. Mancini, G.J.; Pearson, G.J.; Barry, A.R.; Couture, P.; Dayan, N.; Francis, G.A.; Genest, J.; Gregoire, J.C.; Hegele, R.A.; Leiter, L.A. Prevention and Management of Cardiovascular Disease in Primary Care: A Comment on the PEER Simplified Lipid Guideline. *CJC Open* **2024**, *6*, 1189–1198. [CrossRef]
52. Zhu, J.X.; Nash, D.M.; McArthur, E.; Farag, A.; Garg, A.X.; Jain, A.K. Nephrology comanagement and the quality of antibiotic prescribing in primary care for patients with chronic kidney disease: A retrospective cross-sectional study. *Nephrol. Dial. Transplant.* **2019**, *34*, 642–649. [CrossRef]
53. Hoang, P.; Salbu, R.L. Updated nitrofurantoin recommendations in the elderly: A closer look at the evidence. *Consult. Pharm.* **2016**, *31*, 381–384. [CrossRef] [PubMed]
54. Squadrito, F.J.; del Portal, D. Nitrofurantoin. [Updated 2023 May 29]. In *StatPearls [Internet]*; StatPearls Publishing: Treasure Island, FL, USA, 2025; Available online: https://www.ncbi.nlm.nih.gov/books/NBK470526/ (accessed on 11 March 2025).
55. Okoro, R.N.; Farate, V.T. The use of nephrotoxic drugs in patients with chronic kidney disease. *Int. J. Clin. Pharm.* **2019**, *41*, 767–775. [CrossRef]
56. Solak, Y.; Biyik, Z.; Gaipov, A.; Kayrak, M.; Ciray, H.; Cizmecioglu, A.; Tonbul, H.Z.; Turk, S. Drug dose adjustment in dialysis patients admitted in clinics other than internal medicine. *Am. J. Ther.* **2016**, *23*, e68–e73. [CrossRef] [PubMed]
57. Barbieri, M.A.; Rottura, M.; Cicala, G.; Mandraffino, R.; Marino, S.; Irrera, N.; Mannucci, C.; Santoro, D.; Squadrito, F.; Arcoraci, V. Chronic kidney disease management in general practice: A focus on inappropriate drugs prescriptions. *J. Clin. Med.* **2020**, *9*, 1346. [CrossRef] [PubMed]
58. MacRae, C.; Mercer, S.; Guthrie, B. Potentially inappropriate primary care prescribing in people with chronic kidney disease: A cross-sectional analysis of a large population cohort. *Br. J. Gen. Pract.* **2021**, *71*, e483–e490. [CrossRef]
59. Silva-Almodóvar, A.; Hackim, E.; Wolk, H.; Nahata, M.C. Potentially inappropriately prescribed medications among Medicare medication therapy management eligible patients with chronic kidney disease: An observational analysis. *J. Gen. Intern. Med.* **2021**, *36*, 2346–2352. [CrossRef]
60. Zuber, K.; Liles, A.M.; Davis, J. Medication dosing in patients with chronic kidney disease. *JAAPA* **2013**, *26*, 19–25. [CrossRef]
61. Deed, G.; Ackermann, E.; Arthur, I.; Barlow, J.; Jagadeesan, S.; Kawol, D.; Kilov, G.; Leow, S.; Manski-Nankervis, J.-A.; Rasalam, R. *General Practice Management of Type 2 Diabetes: 2016–18. Royal Australian College of General Practitioners (RACGP)*; RACGP: East Melbourne, VIC, Australia, 2016.
62. Alhumaid, S.; Bezabhe, W.M.; Williams, M.; Peterson, G.M. Trends in renal function testing in patients with dementia: A repeated cross-sectional analysis in Australian general practice. *J. Nephrol.* **2025**, 1–9. [CrossRef]

63. Barmano, N.; Walfridsson, U.; Walfridsson, H.; Karlsson, J.-E. Structured care of patients with atrial fibrillation improves guideline adherence. *J. Atr. Fibrillation* **2016**, *9*, 1498. [CrossRef] [PubMed]
64. Brieger, D.; Amerena, J.; Attia, J.R.; Bajorek, B.; Chan, K.H.; Connell, C.; Freedman, B.; Ferguson, C.; Hall, T.; Haqqani, H.M. National Heart Foundation of Australia and Cardiac Society of Australia and New Zealand: Australian clinical guidelines for the diagnosis and management of atrial fibrillation 2018. *Med. J. Aust.* **2018**, *209*, 356–362. [CrossRef] [PubMed]
65. Lip, G.Y.; Lane, D.A. Stroke prevention in atrial fibrillation: A systematic review. *JAMA* **2015**, *313*, 1950–1962. [CrossRef]
66. Bezabhe, W.M.; Bereznicki, L.R.; Radford, J.; Wimmer, B.C.; Curtain, C.; Salahudeen, M.S.; Peterson, G.M. Factors influencing oral anticoagulant use in patients newly diagnosed with atrial fibrillation. *Eur. J. Clin. Investig.* **2021**, *51*, e13457. [CrossRef]
67. Kefale, A.T.; Bezabhe, W.M.; Peterson, G.M. Oral anticoagulant use in patients with atrial fibrillation at low risk of stroke and associated bleeding complications. *J. Clin. Med.* **2023**, *12*, 6182. [CrossRef] [PubMed]
68. Kefale, B.; Peterson, G.M.; Mirkazemi, C.; Dwyer, N.B.; Salahudeen, M.S.; Radford, J.; Boland, C.M.; Bezabhe, W.M. Does hospitalisation improve oral anticoagulant optimisation in patients with atrial fibrillation? *Eur. J. Clin. Investig.* **2025**, *55*, e70011. [CrossRef]
69. Tesfaye, W.H.; Castelino, R.L.; Wimmer, B.C.; Zaidi, S.T.R. Inappropriate prescribing in chronic kidney disease: A systematic review of prevalence, associated clinical outcomes and impact of interventions. *Int. J. Clin. Pract.* **2017**, *71*, e12960. [CrossRef]

Journal of
Clinical Medicine

MDPI

Article

Muscle Quality Assessed by the Phase Angle Can Predict Renal Prognosis in Patients with Chronic Kidney Disease

Yukari Mae, Tomoaki Takata *, Sosuke Taniguchi, Kana Kageyama, Yudai Fujino, Shotaro Hoi, Takuji Iyama and Hajime Isomoto

Division of Gastroenterology and Nephrology, Faculty of Medicine, Tottori University, Yonago, Tottori 683-8504, Japan
* Correspondence: t-takata@tottori-u.ac.jp; Tel.: +81-859-38-6527

Abstract: Background/Objectives: Muscle quality reflects functional characteristics beyond muscle mass and may offer prognostic insights in patients with chronic kidney disease (CKD). This study investigated whether muscle quality predicts sarcopenia and renal outcomes in non-dialysis CKD patients. **Methods**: We prospectively recruited 93 patients with CKD (stage G1–5). Muscle quality was evaluated using phase angle (PhA) derived from bioelectrical impedance analysis. Sarcopenia was diagnosed based on criteria from the Asian Working Group for Sarcopenia. The primary renal outcome was defined as a > 30% decline in eGFR or the initiation of dialysis. Logistic regression identified factors associated with sarcopenia. Kaplan–Meier and Cox regression analyses were used to assess predictors of renal outcomes. **Results**: Lower PhA (odds ratio [OR] 0.044, $p = 0.002$) and BMI (OR 0.648, $p = 0.015$) were independently associated with sarcopenia. Sex-specific PhA cutoffs of 4.50° for men and 4.00° for women yielded high diagnostic accuracy for sarcopenia (AUC: 0.878 and 0.969, respectively). Over a median observation period of 574 days, patients with lower PhA values showed a significantly higher risk of poor renal outcomes, independent of confounding factors (hazard ratio [HR] 4.540, $p = 0.011$), even after adjustment for age, sex, BMI, systolic blood pressure, diastolic blood pressure, eGFR, and albumin. However, muscle mass was not significantly associated with renal prognosis. **Conclusions**: PhA is a non-invasive marker that may reflect muscle quality and is associated with sarcopenia and renal outcomes in CKD. It may help inform risk stratification in clinical practice.

Keywords: bioelectrical impedance analysis; chronic kidney disease; muscle quality; phase angle; sarcopenia; renal prognosis

1. Introduction

The global burden of chronic kidney disease (CKD) is escalating, particularly due to its high prevalence among aging populations. This trend poses a growing challenge to healthcare systems worldwide [1]. Patients with CKD often have various comorbidities, such as cardiovascular diseases, mineral bone disorders, and sarcopenia. The characteristic pathophysiology of CKD, such as uremic toxin accumulation, malnutrition, metabolic abnormality, and inflammation, can negatively affect skeletal muscle by altering its composition and function [2–4], leading to sarcopenia. Assessment of sarcopenia in clinical practice is necessary because it is strongly associated with quality of life and can influence the evaluation of renal function [5]. Furthermore, sarcopenia can be a risk factor for further decline in renal function and is associated with increased mortality in patients with CKD [6–10]. The close interplay between CKD and sarcopenia in a vicious cycle underscores the importance of early and accurate assessment of sarcopenia in patients with CKD.

Traditionally, sarcopenia is diagnosed based on muscle mass and strength [11]. However, recent consensus highlights the importance of muscle quality, which reflects the structural and functional integrity of muscle beyond quantity alone [12,13]. Muscle quality is thought to deteriorate earlier than muscle mass and may thus serve as a more sensitive indicator of early-stage sarcopenia [12,13]. Despite its clinical relevance, evaluating muscle quality remains challenging due to the need for imaging modalities such as magnetic resonance imaging (MRI) or dual-energy X-ray absorptiometry (DXA), which are often impractical in routine clinical settings. Bioelectrical impedance analysis (BIA) serves as a practical and non-intrusive tool for analyzing body composition. One key parameter derived from BIA is the phase angle (PhA), which is calculated as the arctangent of the ratio of reactance (Xc) to resistance (R). When an alternating current flows through the human body, intact cell membranes act as capacitors, delaying the current and causing a phase shift between the voltage and current. This time lag, resulting from the capacitive properties of cell membranes and tissue interfaces, is expressed as the PhA. A higher PhA generally indicates better cellular health and function, whereas a lower PhA suggests impaired membrane integrity or reduced cell mass. Specifically, a decrease in PhA reflects a reduction in Xc—primarily due to compromised cell membrane integrity or a decline in myocyte number—and is often accompanied by an increase in R caused by fatty infiltration of muscle tissue. This combination of decreased Xc and increased R indicates a deterioration in muscle quality [14–16]. Recent studies have demonstrated a positive correlation between muscle quality, defined as grip strength (HGS) relative to arm muscle mass, and PhA, supporting its use as a surrogate marker of muscle quality [16]. Prior studies have demonstrated associations between PhA and muscle function, nutritional status, inflammation, and mortality, particularly in patients on maintenance hemodialysis [17–21]. However, the clinical usefulness of PhA in evaluating sarcopenia and predicting renal prognosis in patients with CKD who are not undergoing dialysis has not been fully explored.

The objectives of this study were to (1) investigate the association between muscle quality and sarcopenia in individuals with CKD, (2) identify sex-specific PhA thresholds for sarcopenia detection, and (3) assess the predictive value of muscle quality for renal outcomes.

2. Materials and Methods

2.1. Study Population and Design

This single-center prospective study was conducted at the Department of Nephrology, Tottori University Hospital (Yonago, Japan). Patients were prospectively enrolled between April 2021 and October 2022, and each patient was followed up for renal outcomes until March 2025 or the occurrence of a renal event, whichever came first. The inclusion criteria were as follows: diagnosis of CKD and provision of written informed consent. CKD was defined as an estimated glomerular filtration rate (eGFR) < 60 mL/min/1.73 m^2 [22] or a urine protein-to-creatinine ratio (UPCR) > 0.15 g/gCr for a period exceeding 3 months. Therefore, this definition encompasses CKD stages G1 to G5, incorporating both early-stage patients with proteinuria and those with reduced eGFR. Among 131 patients initially enrolled, 38 who met the exclusion criteria—age < 20 years, current dialysis treatment, insufficient data for sarcopenia diagnosis, or presence of implanted medical devices—were excluded, resulting in 93 patients for final analysis. Patients were followed up until March 2025, and their renal outcome, defined as a > 30% reduction in the eGFR or initiation of dialysis, was recorded [23,24]. All participants provided written informed consent prior to enrollment. The study protocol adhered to the principles of the Declaration of Helsinki and was reviewed and approved by the Ethics Committee of Tottori University Hospital (Approval No. 20A186).

2.2. Body Composition Analysis and Sarcopenia Diagnosis

Body composition measurements were conducted 30–60 min before non-fasting blood collection. Height was measured using a height meter (Seca 228; Seka Nihon, Chiba, Japan). Body mass index (BMI) was calculated by dividing the body weight by the square of height. Muscle mass was evaluated by assessing the appendicular skeletal muscle mass (ASM) and skeletal muscle mass index (SMI) was calculated by dividing the ASM by the square of the height (kg/m^2). Muscle quality was assessed by PhA using MC-780A-N (TANITA, Tokyo, Japan). PhA was automatically calculated by the device from the resistance (R) and reactance (Xc) values obtained at 50 kHz using the following formula: PhA (°) = arctangent (Xc/R) × (180/π). Handgrip strength (HGS) was measured using a digital grip strength meter (GRIP-D; TAKEI, Niigata, Japan), and the maximum value among two repetitive measurements was used. Blood pressure was measured in the seated position after at least 5 min of rest using an automated sphygmomanometer. Blood pressure measurements were successfully obtained for all patients, with no missing data. Two consecutive readings were obtained, and the average values were recorded as systolic and diastolic blood pressure, respectively. Sarcopenia was assessed using HGS and skeletal muscle mass index (SMI), based on the recommendations of the European Working Group on Sarcopenia in Older People (EWGSOP) [11] and the Asian Working Group for Sarcopenia (AWGS) [25]. Diagnostic cutoff values for HGS and SMI were adopted from the AWGS criteria, with sarcopenia defined as HGS <26 kg for men and <18 kg for women, and SMI <7.0 kg/m^2 for men and <5.7 kg/m^2 for women. Blood and intermediate urine samples were collected after the body composition measurements.

2.3. Statistical Analysis

Continuous data were summarized as either mean ± standard deviation or median with range, depending on their distribution. Normality was assessed using the Kolmogorov–Smirnov test. Comparisons of clinical characteristics were conducted between patients with and without sarcopenia; intergroup differences were analyzed using χ^2, Student's t, or Mann–Whitney U tests, depending on their distribution. Because some variables were not normally distributed, the correlations between PhA and clinical parameters—age, BMI, HGS, ASM, eGFR, Alb, and UPCR—were analyzed using Spearman's rank correlation coefficient. Logistic regression analysis was performed to identify the factors associated with sarcopenia. Receiver operating characteristic (ROC) curve analysis was conducted to determine the PhA cutoff value for detecting sarcopenia, and the optimal cutoff was identified using the Youden index. Kaplan–Meier survival analysis and the Log-rank test were used to compare renal outcomes between the two groups. Additionally, Cox proportional hazards regression analyses were conducted to assess factors contributing to renal outcomes. To account for nutritional status, serum albumin was included as a covariate in the Cox regression model. In both univariate and multivariate Cox regression analyses, systolic and diastolic blood pressures were also included as covariates, as blood pressure is a clinically important factor influencing renal prognosis. Variables included in the multivariate model were selected based on clinical relevance and statistical significance in univariate analysis ($p < 0.10$), except for HGS, which was excluded due to its close correlation with PhA to avoid multicollinearity. Statistical analyses were performed using Stat-Flex (version 6.0 for Windows, Artec, Osaka, Japan). Statistical significance was set at $p < 0.05$.

3. Results

3.1. Patient Characteristics

Of the 131 patients initially enrolled, 38 did not meet the inclusion criteria or were otherwise excluded, resulting in 93 patients being analyzed. The cohort comprised 59 male and 34 female participants, with a median age of 67.0 years (range: 26.0–89.0), as shown in Table 1. The eGFR was 42.7 (4.8–114.3) mL/min/1.73 m^2. Body mass index (BMI) was 23.9 ± 4.1 kg/m^2, systolic blood pressure (sBP) was 135.0 (103.0–185.0) mmHg, diastolic blood pressure (dBP) was 81.0 (45.0–102.0) mmHg, HGS was 26.9 (8.1–58.5) kg, SMI was 7.39 (5.13–10.88) kg/m^2, PhA was 5.13 ± 0.9°, Alb was 3.90 (2.3–4.8) g/dL, and UPCR was 0.65 (0.01–11.53). Eleven patients (six men and five women) had sarcopenia. The sarcopenia group consisted of older individuals (81.5 [29.0–89.0] years), compared with the non-sarcopenia group (66.0 [26.0–84.0] years, p = 0.002). Additionally, the sarcopenia group showed significantly lower height (1.53 ± 0.09 m vs. 1.63 ± 0.09 m, $p < 0.001$), body weight (51.7 [34.1–58.1] kg vs. 62.9 [43.7–102.9] kg, $p < 0.001$), BMI (20.5 ± 3.6 kg/m^2 vs. 24.3 ± 4.0 kg/m^2, p = 0.005), HGS (14.0 [8.1–26.4] kg vs. 28.3 [11.1–58.5] kg, $p < 0.001$), ASM (13.7 ± 2.6 kg vs. 21.1 ± 4.5 kg, $p < 0.001$), SMI (5.56 [5.13–6.49] kg/m^2 vs. 7.73 [6.04–10.88] kg/m^2, $p < 0.001$), and PhA (3.87 ± 0.6° vs. 5.28 ± 0.9°, $p < 0.001$), compared with the non-sarcopenia group.

Table 1. Characteristics of the participants in the study groups.

Parameter	Non-Sarcopenia Group (n = 82)	Sarcopenia Group (n = 11)	p Value
Age (years)	66.0 (26.0–84.0)	81.5 (29.0–89.0)	0.002
Sex (male/female)	53/29	6/5	
Cause of renal disease			
Glomerulonephritis	43.4%	54.5%	
Diabetic nephropathy	18.1%	0%	
Nephrosclerosis	6.0%	27.3%	
Tubulointerstitial nephritis	6.0%	0%	
Polycystic kidney disease	3.6%	0%	
Other/unknown	22.9%	18.2%	
Height (m)	1.63 ± 0.09	1.53 ± 0.09	<0.001
Body weight (kg)	62.9 (43.7–102.9)	51.7 (34.1–58.1)	<0.001
BMI (kg/m^2)	24.3 ± 4.0	20.5 ± 3.6	0.005
sBP (mmHg)	134.5 (103.0–102.0)	142.0 (110.0–173.0)	0.111
dBP (mmHg)	81 (45.0–185.0)	76 (68.0–91.0)	0.730
HGS (kg)	28.3 (11.1–58.5)	14.0 (8.1–26.4)	<0.001
ASM (kg)	21.1 ± 4.5	13.7 ± 2.6	<0.001
SMI (kg/m^2)	7.73 (6.04–10.88)	5.56 (5.13–6.49)	<0.001
PhA (°)	5.28 ± 0.9	3.87 ± 0.6	<0.001
eGFR (mL/min/1.73 m^2)	42.7 (4.8–114.3)	45.8 (21.3–85.9)	0.916
Alb (g/dL)	3.90 (2.3–4.8)	3.70 (3.3–4.5)	0.142
UPCR (g/gCr)	0.67 (0.01–11.53)	0.45 (0.04–2.81)	0.382
CKD stage			
G1–2	25.6%	27.3%	
G3a	18.3%	27.3%	
G3b	26.8%	18.2%	

Table 1. *Cont.*

Parameter	Non-Sarcopenia Group (n = 82)	Sarcopenia Group (n = 11)	p Value
G4	20.7%	27.3%	
G5	8.5%	0%	

BMI; body mass index, sBP; systolic blood pressure, dBP; diastolic blood pressure, HGS; handgrip strength, ASM; appendicular skeletal muscle, SMI; skeletal muscle, PhA; phase angle, eGFR; estimated glomerular filtration rate, Alb; albumin, UPCR; urine protein-to-creatinine ratio, CKD; chronic kidney disease. Values are presented as mean ± standard deviation (standard deviation), median (range), and percentage. Data are presented as mean ± standard deviation (SD) for normally distributed variables, median (range) for non-normally distributed variables, and percentages for categorical variables. Intergroup comparisons between sarcopenia and non-sarcopenia groups were performed using Student's t-test or Mann–Whitney U test for continuous variables, depending on their distribution, and χ^2 test for categorical variables.

3.2. Correlation Between PhA and Clinical Variables

A correlation analysis using Spearman's rank correlation coefficient revealed that PhA was significantly associated with multiple clinical parameters. PhA demonstrated a strong negative correlation with age (r = −0.615, $p < 0.001$) and strong positive correlations with HGS (r = 0.629, $p < 0.001$) and ASM (r = 0.555, $p < 0.001$). Moderate positive correlations were also observed between PhA and eGFR (r = 0.388, $p < 0.001$) and Alb (r = 0.338, $p < 0.001$). The correlation between PhA and BMI was weaker and did not reach statistical significance (r = 0.192, $p = 0.065$). No significant correlation was observed between PhA and UPCR (r = −0.254, $p = 0.114$). These findings support the association of PhA with muscle strength, nutritional status, and renal function.

3.3. Factors Associated with Sarcopenia

In univariate logistic regression analysis, sarcopenia was coded as 1 and non-sarcopenia as 0 in the dependent variable. Age (odds ratio [OR]: 1.070, 95% confidence interval [CI]: 1.007–1.137, $p = 0.029$), BMI (OR: 0.736, 95% CI: 0.586–0.924, p = 0. 008), HGS (OR: 0.809, 95% CI: 0.713–0.918, $p < 0.001$), ASM (OR: 0.550, 95% CI: 0.389–0.777, $p <$ 0.001), and PhA (OR: 0.120, 95% CI: 0.038–0.379, $p < 0.001$) were associated with sarcopenia (Table 2). We further conducted multivariate logistic regression analysis to investigate the factors contributing to sarcopenia. Given that muscle strength and mass are included in the diagnostic criteria for sarcopenia and are strongly associated with each other, parameters reflecting them, such as HGS and ASM, were excluded from the explanatory variables to avoid multicollinearity. We performed binary logistic regression analysis, including age, sex, BMI, and PhA as explanatory variables, showing that BMI (OR: 0.648, 95% CI: 0.457–0.918, $p = 0.015$) and the PhA (OR: 0.044, 95% CI: 0.006–0.316, $p = 0.002$) were independently associated with sarcopenia (Table 2).

Table 2. Factors associated with sarcopenia.

Parameter	Univariate		Multivariate	
	Odds Ratio (95% CI)	p Value	Odds Ratio (95% CI)	p Value
Age	1.070 (1.007–1.137)	0.029	0.979 (0.910–1.052)	0.558
Sex (Ref. M)	1.523 (0.428–5.424)	0.516	0.267 (0.039–1.822)	0.178
BMI	0.736 (0.586–0.924)	0.008	0.648 (0.457–0.918)	0.015
eGFR	1.003 (0.978–1.030)	0.799		
HGS	0.809 (0.713–0.918)	<0.001		
ASM	0.550 (0.389–0.777)	<0.001		
PhA	0.120 (0.038–0.379)	<0.001	0.044 (0.006–0.316)	0.002

CI; confidence interval, Ref; reference, M; male, BMI; body mass index, eGFR; estimated glomerular filtration rate, HGS; handgrip strength, ASM; appendicular skeletal muscle, PhA; phase angle. Univariate and multivariate logistic regression analyses were performed to identify factors associated with sarcopenia. Odds ratios and 95% CI were calculated. Variables included in the multivariate model were selected based on clinical relevance and absence of multicollinearity.

3.4. Diagnostic Performance of the PhA for Sarcopenia

ROC curve analysis revealed that the PhA could detect sarcopenia, with an area under the curve (AUC) of 0.878 for men and 0.969 for women (Figure 1). Using Youden's index, we identified the optimal PhA thresholds as 4.50° in men and 4.00° in women. These values corresponded to sensitivity/specificity rates of 85.2%/80.0% and 89.7%/100.0%, respectively. A statistical comparison of AUCs between sexes was not performed in this study. These findings indicate that the PhA has a high diagnostic ability for sarcopenia.

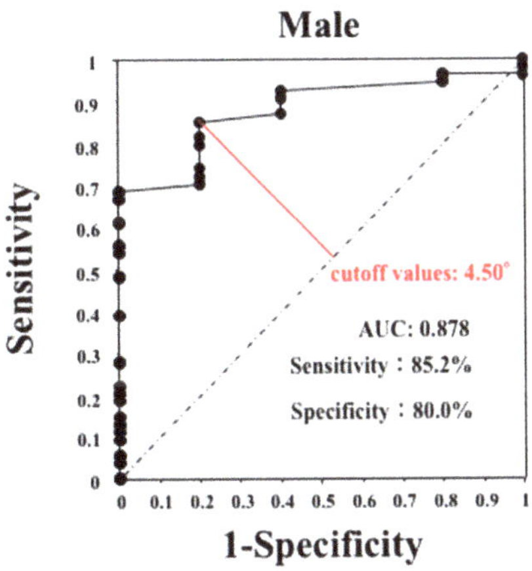

(a)

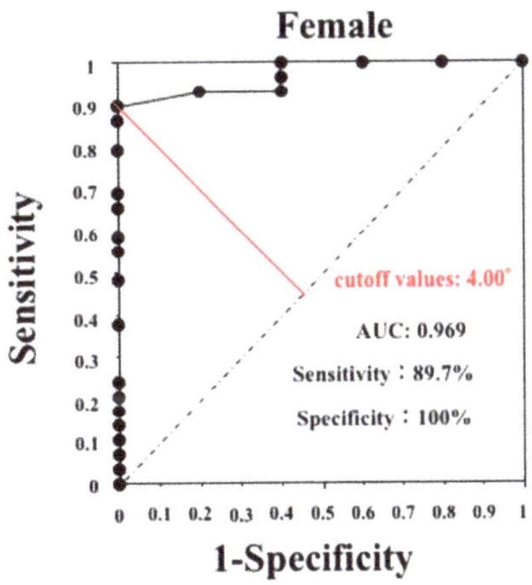

(b)

Figure 1. The ROC curve of PhA to detect sarcopenia. (**a**) The ROC curve for men showing an AUC of 0.878 with a cutoff value of 4.50° (sensitivity: 85.2%, specificity: 80.0%). (**b**) The ROC curve for women showing an AUC of 0.969 with a cutoff value of 4.00° (sensitivity: 89.7%, specificity: 100%). The optimal cutoff values were determined using Youden's index. AUC: area under the curve, ROC: receiver operating characteristic, PhA: phase angle.

3.5. Impact of the PhA on Renal Prognosis

Next, we investigated whether low PhA and the presence of sarcopenia could predict renal outcomes in patients with CKD. During a median follow-up period of 574 days, 21 patients experienced a > 30% decline in eGFR or initiated dialysis. To assess the predictive value of PhA, the patients were divided into "low" and "high" PhA groups based on the sex-specific cutoff values established from the ROC curve analysis (4.50° for men and 4.00° for women). Kaplan–Meier curve analysis revealed that patients with low PhA demonstrated a significantly poor prognosis, compared with those with high PhA ($p < 0.001$) (Figure 2a). During the follow-up period, renal events occurred in 12 patients (48.0%) in the low PhA group and in 9 patients (13.2%) in the high PhA group, further supporting the prognostic significance of PhA. In contrast, when the patients were divided based on the presence of sarcopenia, renal prognosis did not differ between the groups (Figure 2b).

We further conducted Cox regression analysis to assess the risk factors for renal outcomes. In the univariate model using PhA as a continuous variable, age (hazard ratio [HR]: 1.039, 95% CI: 1.004–1.075, $p = 0.029$), eGFR (HR: 0.923, 95% CI: 0.891–0.957, $p < 0.001$), Alb (HR: 0.215, 95% CI: 0.091–0.508, $p < 0.001$), and PhA (HR: 0.395, 95% CI: 0.235–0.665, $p < 0.001$) were significantly associated with renal outcomes. Neither sBP (HR: 1.015, 95% CI: 0.986–1.046, $p = 0.315$) nor dBP (HR: 0.966, 95% CI: 0.931–1.003, $p = 0.069$) was significantly associated with renal outcomes. In the multivariate model, adjusted for age, sex, BMI, sBP, dBP, eGFR, and Alb, PhA remained an independent predictor of renal outcomes (HR:

0.400, 95% CI: 0.190–0.843, $p = 0.016$), while Alb lost statistical significance (HR: 0.448, 95% CI: 0.150–1.335, $p = 0.150$) (Table 3). In addition, we performed a separate analysis using PhA as a dichotomous variable, based on the sex-specific cutoff values identified through ROC analysis (4.50° for men and 4.00° women). Patients with low PhA showed a significantly higher risk of renal events compared with those with high PhA (HR: 4.540, 95% CI: 1.417–14.54, $p = 0.011$) (Table 4). This analysis was conducted to evaluate the prognostic utility of the established cutoff values.

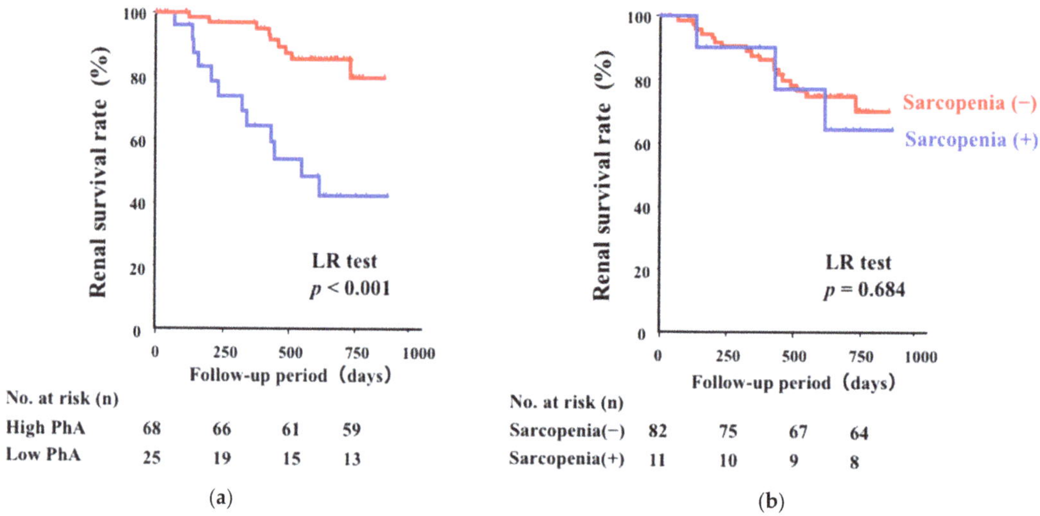

Figure 2. The Kaplan–Meier survival curves for renal outcomes. (**a**) The patients were divided based on their PhA. The renal survival was significantly lower in patients with low PhA (Log-rank test, $p < 0.001$). (**b**) The patients were divided based on the presence of sarcopenia. No significant difference in renal survival was observed between the groups (Log-rank test, $p = 0.684$). PhA; phase angle, LR test; Log-rank test.

Table 3. Cox hazard ratios for renal outcomes.

Parameter	Univariate		Multivariate	
	HR (95% CI)	*p* Value	HR (95% CI)	*p* Value
Age	1.039 (1.004–1.075)	0.029	0.987 (0.944–1.032)	0.563
Sex (Ref. M)	0.838 (0.347–2.025)	0.695	0.413 (0.142–1.199)	0.104
BMI	0.999 (0.901–1.108)	0.987	0.977 (0.873–1.093)	0.637
sBP	1.015 (0.986–1.046)	0.315	0.982 (0.945–1.022)	0.376
dBP	0.966 (0.931–1.003)	0.069	1.002 (0.959–1.047)	0.929
eGFR	0.923 (0.891–0.957)	<0.001	0.929 (0.893–0.966)	<0.001
Alb	0.215 (0.091–0.508)	<0.001	0.448 (0.150–1.335)	0.150
HGS	0.955 (0.911–1.001)	0.057		
ASM	1.010 (0.918–1.111)	0.838		
PhA	0.395 (0.235–0.665)	<0.001	0.400 (0.190–0.843)	0.016

HR; hazard ratio, CI; confidence interval, Ref; reference, M; male, BMI; body mass index, sBP; systolic blood pressure, dBP; diastolic blood pressure, eGFR; estimated glomerular filtration rate, Alb; albumin, HGS; handgrip strength, ASM; appendicular skeletal muscle, PhA; phase angle. Univariate and multivariate Cox proportional hazards regression analyses were conducted to evaluate factors associated with renal outcomes. HR and 95% CI were calculated. Variables included in the multivariate model were selected based on clinical relevance and statistical significance ($p < 0.10$) in the univariate analysis. To avoid multicollinearity with PhA, HGS was excluded from the multivariate analysis.

Table 4. Cox proportional hazards analysis for renal outcomes using dichotomized PhA values.

Parameter	Multivariate	
	HR (95% CI)	***p* Value**
Age	0.990 (0.947–1.034)	0.646
Sex (Ref. M)	0.783 (0.290–2.114)	0.630
BMI	0.981 (0.882–1.092)	0.728
sBP	0.976 (0.937–1.017)	0.253
dBP	1.005 (0.958–1.054)	0.844
eGFR	0.921 (0.884–0.959)	<0.001
Alb	0.557 (0.190–1.636)	0.287
High PhA	Ref.	–
Low PhA	4.540 (1.417–14.54)	0.011

HR, hazard ratio; CI, confidence interval; Ref, reference; M; male, BMI; body mass index, sBP; systolic blood pressure, dBP; diastolic blood pressure, eGFR; estimated glomerular filtration rate, Alb; albumin, PhA; phase angle. Cox proportional hazards regression analysis was conducted using sex-specific PhA cutoff values derived from ROC analysis (4.50° for men, 4.00° for women). PhA was entered as a dichotomous variable, with the high PhA group set as the reference. HR and 95% CI were calculated to assess the risk of renal outcomes in patients with low PhA.

4. Discussion

This study demonstrated that PhA was significantly associated with both sarcopenia and renal prognosis in patients with CKD. We established the optimal PhA cutoff values for identifying sarcopenia in both sexes. Furthermore, we revealed that patients with low PhA were at a higher risk of poor renal prognosis, compared with those with high PhA. These findings highlight the clinical significance of PhA in the management of patients with CKD.

PhA reflects cell integrity [26,27], muscle condition [28,29], nutritional status [30,31], and inflammation [32]. As PhA reflects alterations in muscle components, it may be an early indicator of sarcopenia. This study revealed that low BMI and PhA were associated with sarcopenia in non-dialysis patients with CKD. Notably, PhA is strongly associated with sarcopenia. This study demonstrated that the OR of the PhA for sarcopenia was 0.044, indicating every 1° decrease in PhA increased the risk of sarcopenia by 22.7 times. This increase is remarkable when compared with the previous reports in patients on maintenance hemodialysis, in which every 1° decrease in PhA was associated with a 1.96 to 4.17 times increase in the risk of sarcopenia [17,18,20,21]. Given that muscle mass and function tend to be preserved in patients not on maintenance dialysis compared with those undergoing dialysis [7,33–35], PhA may serve as an early indicator of potential sarcopenia. We also observed that BMI was associated with the higher risk for sarcopenia. Previous studies in patients undergoing hemodialysis have shown that a 1 kg/m^2 increase in BMI reduces the risk of sarcopenia by 26–34% [18,36] which is in line with the OR of BMI for sarcopenia observed in the present study.

In this study, PhA accurately detected sarcopenia in both sexes. We determined the PhA cutoff values for diagnosing sarcopenia: 4.50° for men and 4.00° for women. In an observational study conducted in an Asian population, the PhA was 6.55 ± 1.10° in healthy individuals. Previous studies have reported PhAs of 5.95° for young men, 5.04° for older men, 5.02° for young women, and 4.20° for older women [16]. These observations indicate that the PhA reference values may differ according to sex. Moreover, in patients on maintenance hemodialysis, PhAs of 6.20° [17] and 4.67° [18] in men and 5.70° [17] and 4.60° [18] in women predicted sarcopenia; thus, the PhA cutoff values for diagnosing sarcopenia may differ according to the patients' comorbidities.

Importantly, our study demonstrated that PhA is a significant predictor of renal prognosis in patients with CKD. In univariate Cox regression analysis, PhA showed the strongest association with long-term renal outcomes compared to HGS and ASM, which exhibited only weak correlations. We further adjusted for potential confounders including age, sex, BMI, eGFR, serum albumin, and both systolic and diastolic blood pressure in the multivariate Cox regression model. Notably, neither systolic nor diastolic blood pressure was significantly associated with renal outcomes. Among all variables, only PhA remained independently associated with renal outcomes (HR: 4.540, 95% CI: 1.417–14.54, p = 0.011), whereas serum albumin lost statistical significance (HR: 0.557, 95% CI: 0.190–1.636, p = 0.287). These findings raise the possibility that PhA could provide complementary prognostic information to traditional nutritional and cardiovascular markers, potentially reflecting aspects of muscle cell membrane integrity and muscle quality. Kaplan–Meier analysis also demonstrated that patients with low PhA showed significantly poorer renal outcomes during follow-up, whereas no significant difference in long-term renal outcomes was observed between patients with or without sarcopenia. This lack of association may be partly attributed to the clinical characteristics of the study population. Notably, none of the patients classified as having sarcopenia had diabetic nephropathy (DN), whereas the subgroup with low PhA but without sarcopenia included a higher proportion of patients with DN. Since DN is a leading cause of CKD progression and may be associated with declines in muscle quality even in the absence of marked reductions in muscle mass or strength, PhA may more sensitively detect subtle muscle alterations linked to renal prognosis in these patients. Based on these findings that PhA potentially serves as an accurate and early indicator of renal survival in patients with CKD, we propose to incorporate muscle quality in addition to muscle mass in the assessment of sarcopenia.

Although this study suggests the relevance of muscle quality in diagnosing sarcopenia and predicting renal outcomes in patients with CKD, it has some limitations. First, it was conducted at a single center with a relatively modest sample size (n = 93), which may limit the generalizability of the findings. Moreover, this study analyzed the association between PhA and renal outcomes based on a single baseline measurement; longitudinal changes in PhA during the follow-up period were not assessed. As PhA may fluctuate with changes in muscle quality and overall health status, serial measurements could provide deeper insights into the dynamic relationship between muscle condition and renal prognosis. Future studies incorporating repeated PhA assessments are warranted to clarify these associations and to complement the limitations related to sample size and study design. In addition, although the primary causes of CKD differed between the sarcopenia and non-sarcopenia groups, urinary protein levels did not significantly differ. The degree of renal pathological damage was not available for all patients and thus was not included in the analysis. These factors are important determinants of CKD progression and should be incorporated in future studies to better elucidate the impact of sarcopenia on renal outcomes. Additionally, treatment strategies to prevent CKD progression may vary across institutions and individual patients, potentially influencing renal outcomes. Furthermore, since estimated glomerular filtration rate (eGFR) is calculated from serum creatinine, which is influenced by muscle mass, the presence of sarcopenia may lead to an overestimation of renal function. Although we used established equations and accounted for confounders, this potential bias should be acknowledged when interpreting the results. However, despite the limited number of subjects, associations between PhA and both sarcopenia and renal prognosis were robust, with large effect sizes and relatively narrow confidence intervals. Therefore, our observation is considered clinically relevant. Nevertheless, further multicenter studies with larger, more diverse populations are warranted to validate and expand upon these results.

5. Conclusions

In conclusion, this study suggests that PhA may be a clinically relevant index to assess muscle quality and is associated with both sarcopenia and renal outcomes in patients with CKD. PhA appears to provide prognostic information beyond muscle mass and strength. While these findings indicate a potential role for PhA in risk stratification, further large-scale and multicenter studies are needed to validate its utility in routine clinical practice.

Author Contributions: Conceptualization, Y.M. and T.T.; methodology, Y.M., T.T., S.T., K.K., Y.F., S.H. and T.I.; formal analysis, Y.M.; investigation, T.T.; writing—original draft preparation, Y.M.; writing—review and editing, T.T.; supervision, H.I.; funding acquisition, Y.M. All authors have read and agreed to the published version of the manuscript.

Funding: This study was funded by a Grant-in-Aid for Early-Career Scientists to YM (Japan Society for the Promotion of Science (JSPS) KAKENHI Grant Number JP22K16243) and by a TSUBASA PROJECT to YM (Japanese Society for Dialysis Therapy (JSDT)).

Institutional Review Board Statement: The study was conducted in accordance with the Declaration of Helsinki, and approved by the Ethics Committee of Tottori University Hospital (approval number: 20A186, date of approval: 11 October 2021).

Informed Consent Statement: Informed consent was obtained from all subjects involved in the study.

Data Availability Statement: The data presented in this study are available on request from the corresponding author due to ethical and privacy restrictions, but are available from the corresponding author upon reasonable request.

Conflicts of Interest: The authors declare no conflicts of interest.

References

1. Jager, K.J.; Kovesdy, C.; Langham, R.; Rosenberg, M.; Jha, V.; Zoccali, C. A single number for advocacy and communication—Worldwide more than 850 million individuals have kidney diseases. *Nephrol. Dial. Transplant.* **2019**, *34*, 1803–1805. [CrossRef] [PubMed]
2. Fahal, I.H. Uraemic sarcopenia: Aetiology and implications. *Nephrol. Dial. Transplant.* **2014**, *29*, 1655–1665. [CrossRef]
3. Ishikawa, S.; Naito, S.; Iimori, S.; Takahashi, D.; Zeniya, M.; Sato, H.; Nomura, N.; Sohara, E.; Okado, T.; Uchida, S.; et al. Loop diuretics are associated with greater risk of sarcopenia in patients with non-dialysis-dependent chronic kidney disease. *PLoS ONE* **2018**, *13*, e0192990. [CrossRef] [PubMed]
4. Mae, Y.; Takata, T.; Taniguchi, S.; Fujino, Y.; Kageyama, K.; Hanada, H.; Iyama, T.; Sugihara, T.; Isomoto, H. Selective peroxisome proliferator-activated receptor-α modulator improves hypertriglyceridemia and muscle quality in patients with chronic kidney disease: A retrospective observational study. *Clin. Nutr. ESPEN* **2025**, *65*, 182–188. [CrossRef]
5. Taniguchi, S.; Takata, T.; Mae, Y.; Fujino, Y.; Kageyama, K.; Hanada, H.; Iyama, T.; Isomoto, H. Managing dosage adjustments in pseudo-hypocreatinemia: Insights from vancomycin-induced nephrotoxicity in a sarcopenic patient. *Yonago Acta Med.* **2024**, *67*, 358–362. [CrossRef]
6. Zheng, X.; Ren, X.; Jiang, M.; Han, L.; Zhong, C. Association of Sarcopenia with Rapid Kidney Function Decline and Chronic Kidney Disease in Adults with Normal Kidney Function. *Br. J. Nutr.* **2024**, *131*, 821–828. [CrossRef] [PubMed]
7. Pereira, R.A.; Cordeiro, A.C.; Avesani, C.M.; Carrero, J.J.; Lindholm, B.; Amparo, F.C.; Amodeo, C.; Cuppari, L.; Kamimura, M.A. Sarcopenia in Chronic Kidney Disease on Conservative Therapy: Prevalence and Association with Mortality. *Nephrol. Dial. Transplant.* **2015**, *30*, 1718–1725. [CrossRef] [PubMed]
8. Mori, K.; Nishide, K.; Okuno, S.; Shoji, T.; Emoto, M.; Tsuda, A.; Nakatani, S.; Imanishi, Y.; Ishimura, E.; Yamakawa, T.; et al. Impact of diabetes on sarcopenia and mortality in patients undergoing hemodialysis. *BMC Nephrol.* **2019**, *20*, 105. [CrossRef]
9. Mae, Y.; Takata, T.; Yamada, K.; Hamada, S.; Yamamoto, M.; Iyama, T.; Isomoto, H. Creatinine generation rate can detect sarcopenia in patients with hemodialysis. *Clin. Exp. Nephrol.* **2022**, *26*, 272–277. [CrossRef]
10. Takata, T.; Motoe, A.; Tanida, K.; Taniguchi, S.; Ida, A.; Yamada, K.; Hamada, S.; Ogawa, M.; Yamamoto, M.; Mae, Y.; et al. Feasibility of computed tomography-based assessment of skeletal muscle mass in hemodialysis patients. *J. Nephrol.* **2021**, *34*, 465–471. [CrossRef]

11. Cruz-Jentoft, A.J.; Bahat, G.; Bauer, J.; Boirie, Y.; Bruyère, O.; Cederholm, T.; Cooper, C.; Landi, F.; Rolland, Y.; Sayer, A.A.; et al. Sarcopenia: Revised European consensus on definition and diagnosis. *Age Ageing* **2019**, *48*, 16–31. [CrossRef]
12. McGregor, R.A.; Cameron-Smith, D.; Poppitt, S.D. It Is Not Just Muscle Mass: A Review of Muscle Quality, Composition and Metabolism during Ageing as Determinants of Muscle Function and Mobility in Later Life. *Longev. Healthspan* **2014**, *3*, 9. [CrossRef]
13. Fragala, M.S.; Kenny, A.M.; Kuchel, G.A. Muscle quality in aging: A multi-dimensional approach to muscle functioning with applications for treatment. *Sports Med.* **2015**, *45*, 641–658. [CrossRef]
14. Barbosa-Silva, M.C.; Barros, A.J.; Wang, J.; Heymsfield, S.B.; Pierson, R.N., Jr. Bioelectrical impedance analysis: Population reference values for phase angle by age and sex. *Am. J. Clin. Nutr.* **2005**, *82*, 49–52. [CrossRef]
15. Yamada, Y.; Buehring, B.; Krueger, D.; Anderson, R.M.; Schoeller, D.A.; Binkley, N. Electrical properties assessed by bioelectrical impedance spectroscopy as biomarkers of age-related loss of skeletal muscle quantity and quality. *J. Gerontol. A Biol. Sci. Med. Sci.* **2017**, *72*, 1180–1186. [CrossRef] [PubMed]
16. Akamatsu, Y.; Kusakabe, T.; Arai, H.; Yamamoto, Y.; Nakao, K.; Ikeue, K.; Ishihara, Y.; Tagami, T.; Yasoda, A.; Ishii, K.; et al. Phase angle from bioelectrical impedance analysis is a useful indicator of muscle quality. *J. Cachexia Sarcopenia Muscle* **2022**, *13*, 180–189. [CrossRef]
17. Zeng, Y.; Chen, Y.; Yang, Y.; Qiu, Y.; Fu, P.; Yuan, H. Bioelectrical impedance analysis-derived phase angle predicts possible sarcopenia in patients on maintenance hemodialysis: A retrospective study. *BMC Nephrol.* **2024**, *25*, 357. [CrossRef] [PubMed]
18. Ding, Y.; Chang, L.; Zhang, H.; Wang, S. Predictive value of phase angle in sarcopenia in patients on maintenance hemodialysis. *Nutrition* **2022**, *94*, 111527. [CrossRef]
19. Chen, Y.; Wu, J.; Ran, L.; Yu, D.; Chen, X.; Liu, M. The combination of phase angle and age has a good diagnostic value for sarcopenia in continuous ambulatory peritoneal dialysis patients. *Front. Nutr.* **2022**, *9*, 1036796. [CrossRef] [PubMed]
20. Wang, Y.; Hu, Y.; Zhang, M.; Jin, H.; Wen, Y.; Tang, R.; Wang, B.; Liu, B.; Liu, H. Bioelectrical impedance analysis-derived phase angle predicts sarcopenia in patients on maintenance hemodialysis. *Nutr. Clin. Pract.* **2023**, *38*, 881–888. [CrossRef]
21. Bae, E.; Lee, T.W.; Bae, W.; Kim, S.; Choi, J.; Jang, H.N.; Chang, S.H.; Park, D.J. Impact of phase angle and sarcopenia estimated by bioimpedance analysis on clinical prognosis in patients undergoing hemodialysis: A retrospective study. *Medicine* **2022**, *101*, e29375. [CrossRef]
22. Matsuo, S.; Imai, E.; Horio, M.; Yasuda, Y.; Tomita, K.; Nitta, K.; Yamagata, K.; Tomino, Y.; Yokoyama, H.; Hishida, A.; et al. Revised equations for estimated GFR from serum creatinine in Japan. *Am. J. Kidney Dis.* **2009**, *53*, 982–992. [CrossRef]
23. Coresh, J.; Turin, T.C.; Matsushita, K.; Sang, Y.; Ballew, S.H.; Appel, L.J.; Arima, H.; Chadban, S.J.; Cirillo, M.; Djurdjev, O.; et al. Decline in estimated glomerular filtration rate and subsequent risk of end-stage renal disease and mortality. *JAMA* **2014**, *311*, 2518–2531. [CrossRef]
24. Matsushita, K.; Chen, J.; Sang, Y.; Ballew, S.H.; Shimazaki, R.; Fukagawa, M.; Imai, E.; Coresh, J.; Hishida, A. Risk of end-stage renal disease in Japanese patients with chronic kidney disease increases proportionately to decline in estimated glomerular filtration rate. *Kidney Int.* **2016**, *90*, 1109–1114. [CrossRef] [PubMed]
25. Chen, L.K.; Woo, J.; Assantachai, P.; Auyeung, T.W.; Chou, M.Y.; Iijima, K.; Jang, H.C.; Kang, L.; Kim, M.; Kim, S.; et al. Asian Working Group for Sarcopenia: 2019 Consensus Update on Sarcopenia Diagnosis and Treatment. *J. Am. Med. Dir. Assoc.* **2020**, *21*, 300–307.e2. [CrossRef]
26. Gonzalez, M.C.; Barbosa-Silva, T.G.; Bielemann, R.M.; Gallagher, D.; Heymsfield, S.B. Phase angle and its determinants in healthy subjects: Influence of body composition. *Am. J. Clin. Nutr.* **2016**, *103*, 712–716. [CrossRef]
27. Norman, K.; Stobäus, N.; Pirlich, M.; Bosy-Westphal, A. Bioelectrical phase angle and impedance vector analysis—Clinical relevance and applicability of impedance parameters. *Clin. Nutr.* **2012**, *31*, 854–861. [CrossRef]
28. Beberashvili, I.; Azar, A.; Sinuani, I.; Shapiro, G.; Feldman, L.; Stav, K.; Sandbank, J.; Averbukh, Z. Bioimpedance phase angle predicts muscle function, quality of life and clinical outcome in maintenance hemodialysis patients. *Eur. J. Clin. Nutr.* **2014**, *68*, 683–689. [CrossRef] [PubMed]
29. Basile, C.; Della-Morte, D.; Cacciatore, F.; Gargiulo, G.; Galizia, G.; Roselli, M.; Curcio, F.; Bonaduce, D.; Abete, P. Phase angle as bioelectrical marker to identify elderly patients at risk of sarcopenia. *Exp. Gerontol.* **2014**, *58*, 43–46. [CrossRef] [PubMed]
30. Kyle, U.G.; Soundar, E.P.; Genton, L.; Pichard, C. Can phase angle determined by bioelectrical impedance analysis assess nutritional risk? A comparison between healthy and hospitalized subjects. *Clin. Nutr.* **2012**, *31*, 875–881. [CrossRef]
31. Lukaski, H.C.; Kyle, U.G.; Kondrup, J. Assessment of adult malnutrition and prognosis with bioelectrical impedance analysis: Phase angle and impedance ratio. *Curr. Opin. Clin. Nutr. Metab. Care* **2017**, *20*, 330–339. [CrossRef] [PubMed]
32. Kosacka, M.; Korzeniewska, A.; Jankowska, R. The evaluation of body composition, adiponectin, C-reactive protein and cholesterol levels in patients with obstructive sleep apnea syndrome. *Adv. Clin. Exp. Med.* **2013**, *22*, 817–824. [PubMed]
33. Moon, S.J.; Kim, T.H.; Yoon, S.Y.; Chung, J.H.; Hwang, H.J. Relationship between Stage of Chronic Kidney Disease and Sarcopenia in Korean Aged 40 Years and Older Using the Korea National Health and Nutrition Examination Surveys (KNHANES IV-2, 3, and V-1, 2), 2008–2011. *PLoS ONE* **2015**, *10*, e0130740. [CrossRef]

34. Ren, H.; Gong, D.; Jia, F.; Xu, B.; Liu, Z. Sarcopenia in patients undergoing maintenance hemodialysis: Incidence rate, risk factors and its effect on survival risk. *Ren. Fail.* **2016**, *38*, 364–371. [CrossRef]
35. Kim, J.K.; Choi, S.R.; Choi, M.J.; Kim, S.G.; Lee, Y.K.; Noh, J.W.; Kim, H.J.; Song, Y.R. Prevalence of and factors associated with sarcopenia in elderly patients with end-stage renal disease. *Clin. Nutr.* **2014**, *33*, 64–68. [CrossRef]
36. Hortegal, E.V.F.; Alves, J.J.D.A.; Santos, E.J.F.; Nunes, L.C.R.; da Silva, J.C.G.; Nunes, R.F.; de Almeida Melo, D.; de Carvalho, S.C.R.; da Cunha França, A.K.T.; dos Santos, E.M.; et al. Sarcopenia and inflammation in patients undergoing hemodialysis. *Nutr. Hosp.* **2020**, *37*, 855–862. [PubMed]

Journal of
Clinical Medicine

MDPI

Article

Toward Equitable Kidney Care: Insights from the Survey Among Polish Doctors on the Women's Health in Chronic Kidney Disease Management

Weronika Przybyszewska [1,2], Karol Gawalski [2,3,4], Barbara Bijak [1], Aleksandra Rymarz [1] and Jolanta Małyszko [1,*]

1 Department of Nephrology, Dialysis and Internal Medicine, Medical University of Warsaw, 02-097 Warsaw, Poland; weronika.przybyszewska@wum.edu.pl (W.P.); s083707@student.wum.edu.pl (B.B.); aleksandra.rymarz@wum.edu.pl (A.R.)
2 Doctoral School, Medical University of Warsaw, 02-097 Warsaw, Poland; karol.gawalski@wum.edu.pl
3 Department of Pathology, Military Institute of Medicine, 04-141 Warsaw, Poland
4 Laboratory of Experimental Medicine, Medical University of Warsaw, 02-097 Warsaw, Poland
* Correspondence: jolanta.malyszko@wum.edu.pl

Abstract

Background/Objectives: Chronic kidney disease is more prevalent among women, and there are significant disparities in the management of female patients. Our study aimed to assess the clinical experience and educational needs of physicians in the treatment of reproductive and sex and gender-related health problems in patients with CKD. **Methods:** The three-part survey was distributed among nephrologists and other internal medicine specialists in Poland, both online and in paper form. **Results:** A total of 116 physicians participated in the survey, including 81 nephrologists. Most respondents (64.7%) were female and practiced in multispecialty hospitals (72.4%). While 97.4% managed patients with CKD, only 37.9% reported caring for pregnant women. Experience in sex-specific and pregnancy-related issues was limited—56.9% reported low or minimal experience in managing CKD during pregnancy. Residency training lacked coverage of crucial topics, with 66.2% reporting limited teaching on sex-related CKD progression. Over 90% supported integrating reproductive planning and interdisciplinary care into nephrology, favoring guidelines, conferences, and webinars for education. **Conclusions:** Our study has highlighted a critical discrepancy between the importance of sex-specific and reproductive health considerations in the management of CKD and the current level of clinical experience among Polish doctors.

Keywords: chronic kidney disease; nephrology care; women's health; nephrology education; pregnancy and CKD; gender-related health problems

1. Introduction

Over the last decades, we have been observing a significant increase of about 29.3% in the prevalence and 41.5% in mortality of chronic kidney disease (CKD) [1]. May 2025 marks an important milestone for the entire nephrology society as the WHO (World Health Organization) prioritized CKD within the WHO's noncommunicable diseases (NCD) agenda [2,3]. This historic declaration raises awareness about the burden of kidney diseases, promotes early detection, and motivates actions to guarantee equitable access to care for patients in all communities [4].

According to epidemiological data, CKD is more prevalent among women than men [5]. However, compared to male patients, women are more likely to be offered dialysis at lower estimated glomerular filtration rate (eGFR) levels, are less frequently included on the transplantation lists, and report a lower perceived quality of life. While some of these disparities may be attributed to biological factors, a significant portion stems from diverse socioeconomic influences [6].

As indicated in the Healthy Life in an Urban Setting (HELIUS) study, those biological factors have been widely investigated; however, the impact of sociocultural factors still remains scarce. The research group has found specific gender-related factors that significantly increase the risk of developing kidney diseases. CKD was more common in all women who did little housework, worked part-time or were unemployed, and among men whose financial contribution was equal to their partners' or who were unemployed. This risk could not be explained by other well-known factors contributing to the development of CKD [7]. Nephrologists also increasingly acknowledge the impact of gender disparities in CKD and often perceive women as disadvantaged when faced with kidney disorders. This stems from multiple barriers, including limited access to equitable care, the burden of fulfilling traditional gender roles, and extensive caregiving responsibilities. Women are more vigilant and proactive regarding their health compared to men, which leads to better management of their disease. However, due to many domestic and family-related obligations, as well as concerns about their physical appearance, the time of the initiation of dialysis tends to be delayed compared to male patients [8].

Women at different life stages require a tailored approach to disease management. This need has already been increasingly acknowledged in other medical specialties. For instance, it has also been reflected in the recent Polish hypertension guidelines, which emphasize sex-specific considerations in the management of this chronic disease [9]. Although women's health issues are gaining visibility within the nephrology community [10], there is still a lot more to do to provide equitable care for all female patients. Notably, despite the growing number of breakthrough clinical trials in nephrology, women continue to be underrepresented in clinical trials compared to their actual prevalence of CKD [11]. This may even lead to further implications and greater risk of developing adverse side effects as medication dosing is generally investigated on the groups mostly represented by men [12].

In light of all these data, our study aimed to assess physicians' clinical experience, confidence, and educational needs in managing sex-specific and reproductive health issues in patients with CKD. By surveying doctors across diverse workplace settings, we sought to identify gaps in training and practice, and to explore opportunities for integrating women's health more effectively into nephrology care.

2. Materials and Methods

The study was designed to include both residents and specialists of nephrology and from other fields of internal medicine. The questionnaire was developed following a literature review and subsequently refined through collaborative discussions among the authors. The study has received a positive approval from the Bioethics Committee of the Medical University of Warsaw. The complete survey questionnaire is available in the Supplementary Materials.

The survey consisted of three sections. The first gathered basic demographic information, including gender, years of clinical experience, medical specialty, and workplace setting. To better understand the scope of each respondent's patient population, additional questions addressed average patient age, gender distribution, and employment status.

Section 2 concerned the clinical experience of the participants in the management of patients with CKD, including those undergoing dialysis. Their level of clinical experience

https://doi.org/10.3390/jcm15010196

was assessed using a 5-point Likert scale—from 1 (very low experience), 2 (low experience), 3 (moderate experience), 4 (high experience), to 5 (very high experience).

Further items explored the frequency, using a four-point Likert scale (never, rarely, often, always), with which physicians address women's and reproductive health issues during the process of taking medical history. The survey also investigated the use of ACE-I/ARBs in clinical practice, including prescribing indications and significant reproductive health considerations such as their teratogenic effect.

Section 5 of the survey was directed exclusively to nephrologists, both trainees and certified. A series of Likert scale items was used to evaluate whether sex-specific issues in CKD management (the influence of gender-related factors on disease progression, the impact of CKD, dialysis, and immunosuppressive therapy on fertility, and the management of kidney disorders during pregnancy) are adequately addressed in residency training programs.

Respondents were then asked to self-assess their clinical experience and knowledge across several domains, using a Likert scale from 1 (very low experience), 2 (low experience), 3 (moderate experience), 4 (high experience), to 5 (very high experience). Topics included pregnancy planning in CKD patients and the use of ART in this population.

The survey also gathered nephrologists' views on the need for sex-specific clinical guidelines, the importance of tailoring immunosuppressive therapy to reproductive plans, and the value of interdisciplinary collaboration, including the establishment of referral centers for pregnant patients with CKD. These opinions were measured using a four-point Likert scale (strongly disagree, somewhat disagree, somewhat agree, strongly agree).

Finally, participants were asked to indicate their preferred activities for further education on women's health in nephrology, such as conferences, structured courses, webinars, or clinical guidelines issued by professional societies.

The survey was distributed using a voluntary, anonymous, convenience sampling strategy. The questionnaire was distributed in both paper and digital formats. Printed copies were delivered directly to physicians working in internal medicine and nephrology wards in Warsaw and other hospitals across Poland. The online version, prepared using the Google Forms platform, was disseminated via social media groups dedicated to medical practitioners and circulated through the mailing list of the Polish Society of Nephrology. Because the online distribution channels were open, an exact response rate could not be calculated. Data collection took place between March and July 2025.

Statistical analysis was performed using Statistica software (v13.3, StatSoft, Tulsa, OK, USA). Data expressed on a qualitative scale were presented as the number and percentage. Descriptive statistics were used to summarize demographic characteristics and response distributions. Exploratory subgroup analyses were conducted using the Chi-squared test or Chi-square test with Yates' correction to compare the distributions of these parameters between groups defined by specialty, years of experience, stage of training, and workplace setting. Results were considered statistically significant when $p < 0.05$.

The Microsoft 365 Copilot was used for data analysis and text editing during the preparation of this study.

3. Results

3.1. General Part of the Survey for All Specialists

3.1.1. Demographical Data and Patients' Profile

A total of 116 physicians participated in the survey, including 81 nephrologists, of whom 68 (84%) were certified specialists, and 13 (16%) were trainee doctors. Female respondents comprised the majority, accounting for 64.7% (n = 75) of the sample, while male participants represented 35.3% (n = 41).

https://doi.org/10.3390/jcm15010196

Among all respondents, 76,7% (n = 89) held specialist-level qualifications and nearly 70% (n = 81) reported over 10 years of clinical experience. Residents constituted 23.3% (n = 27) of the sample. In terms of specialization, 81 nephrologists took part in the survey, and 79 reported a background in internal medicine. Other declared specialties included family medicine (n = 4; 3.5%), cardiology (n = 3; 2.6%), and diabetology (n = 1; 0.9%).

The most common workplace setting was a multispecialty hospital (n = 84; 72.4%), followed by specialist outpatient clinics (n = 41; 35.3%) and private healthcare facilities (n = 32; 27.6%). Primary care clinics (n = 16; 3.8%) and municipal or county hospitals (n = 8; 6.9%) were less frequently represented. A detailed summary is presented in Table 1.

Table 1. The characteristics of the respondents' group.

Sex		Number	Percentage
	Female	75	64.66%
	Male	41	35.34%
Years of the clinical experience			
	<5	21	18.10%
	5–10	14	12.07%
	>10	81	69.83%
Stage of professional career			
	Specialist	89	76.72%
	Resident	27	23.28%
Completed or initiated specialization			
	Nephrology	81	69.83%
	Internal medicine	79	68.10%
	Family medicine	4	3.45%
	Cardiology	3	2.59%
	Diabetology	1	0.86%
	Other	36	31.03%
Place(s) of professional employment			
	Multispecialty hospital	84	72.41%
	District/municipal hospital	41	35.34%
	Specialist outpatient practice	32	27.59%
	Primary healthcare practice	16	13.79%
	Non-public (private) facility	8	6.90%

Respondents predominantly cared for older adults, with 76.7% (n = 89) indicating that their patient population was primarily aged 60–80 years. Patients were reported to be almost evenly distributed by gender in 56% (n = 65) of cases, while 21.6% (n = 25) of physicians noted a predominance of female patients. Most patients had completed secondary or vocational education (n = 98; 84.5%), and the vast majority were retired or receiving disability pensions (n = 94; 81.0%).

https://doi.org/10.3390/jcm15010196

The vast majority of respondents (97.4%, n = 113) reported managing patients diagnosed with CKD. Among them, 60.3% (n = 70) estimated that over half of their patient population had CKD, while 26.7% (n = 31) reported a prevalence between 10–50%. Only 10.3% (n = 12) indicated that fewer than 10% of their patients were affected.

A total of 98 physicians (84.5%) reported caring for patients undergoing dialysis. Among patients, hemodialysis was the predominant modality (n = 85; 73.3%), while peritoneal dialysis was reported by only 3.4% of respondents (n = 4).

Only 44 respondents (37.9%) reported providing care to pregnant women in their clinical practice. Among those, the estimated annual number of pregnant patients was generally low: 33.6% (n = 39) cared for fewer than 50 such patients per year, and only 4.3% (n = 5) reported managing more than 50. The patients' profile is summarized in Table 2.

Table 2. The characteristics of the patient population managed by the survey respondents.

Predominant Age Group of Your Patient		**Number**	**Percentage**
	18–40	5	4.31%
	40–60	19	16.38%
	60–80	89	76.72%
	>80	3	2.59%
Estimated predominant sex of patients			
	More or less the same	65	56.04%
	Majority of women	25	21.55%
	Majority of men	12	10.34%
	Difficult to estimate	14	12.07%
Estimated predominant education level of patients			
	Secondary/vocational education	98	88.29%
	Primary education	13	72.22%
	Higher education	5	4.31%
Estimated predominant form of professional activity of patients under care			
	Retired/pensioner	94	83.93%
	Professionally active	19	16.52%
	Student	2	9.09%
	Unemployed	1	0.85%
Patients diagnosed with CKD			
	Yes	113	97.41%
	No	3	2.59%
Estimated percentage of patients with the diagnosis of CKD			
	<10%	12	10.62%
	10–50%	31	27.43%
	>50%	70	61.95%

https://doi.org/10.3390/jcm15010196

Table 2. *Cont.*

Predominant Age Group of Your Patient		Number	Percentage
Patients undergoing dialysis under care			
	Yes	98	84.48%
	No	18	15.52%
Predominant form of dialysis therapy among the patients under care			
	Hemodialysis	85	86.73%
	Peritoneal dialysis	4	4.08%
	More or less the same percentage	9	9.18%
Pregnant patients under your care			
	Yes	44	37.93%
	No	72	62.07%
Estimated number of pregnant patients under care annually			
	<50/year	39	88.64%
	50–100/year	4	9.09%
	>100/year	1	2.27%

3.1.2. Level of the Clinical Experience in the Management of Patients with CKD Across Various Specialties

Respondents across various specialties reported high levels of clinical experience in managing patients with CKD: 58.6% (n = 68), indicating very high, and 13.8% (n = 16) high experience. Moderate experience was reported by 14.7% (n = 17), while only 12.9% (n = 15) described their experience as low or minimal. The higher values of experience level were more frequently reported by physicians with greater experience compared to those with less than 5 years of experience. This association was statistically significant ($p = 0.003$).

Experience in assessing the impact of sex-related factors on kidney disease development was more evenly distributed. Very high experience was reported by only 17.2% (n = 20), high by 19.8% (n = 23), and moderate by 19.8% (n = 23). Low or minimal experience was reported by around 43.1% (n = 50). Among physicians with >10 years of experience, 48.1% (n = 39) reported high or very high experience, while minimal or low experience was most common among those with <5 years (81%, n = 17). This difference was also statistically significant ($p = 0.002$).

Experience in managing kidney diseases related to pregnancy was generally low. Only 6% (n = 7) reported very high experience, and 14.7% (n = 17) high, while 22.4% (n = 26) indicated moderate experience. Minimal or low experience was reported by the majority of doctors—56.9% (n = 66). The association between the years of practice and experience level in this field was also significant ($p = 0.004$).

Regarding the impact of immunosuppressive therapy on fertility, very high experience was reported by 17.2% (n = 20), high by 16.4% (n = 19), and moderate by 22.4% (n = 26). Minimal or low experience was reported by 43.9% (n = 51). Very high experience was reported by 23.5% (n = 19) of physicians with >10 years of practice, compared to 4.8% (n = 1) among those with <5 years.

Similar analysis was also conducted to assess the relationship between the level of expertise and workplace setting. Respondents working in private healthcare facilities reported significantly higher experience in managing CKD ($p = 0.021$) and in assessing sex-related factors in kidney disease development ($p = 0.040$) than those working in other workplaces. Among those employed in private settings, 75% (n = 24) reported very high experience in CKD management, compared to 52.4% (n = 44) outside this setting. Similarly,

https://doi.org/10.3390/jcm15010196

53.1% (n = 17) of private-sector respondents reported high or very high experience in evaluating sex-related factors, compared to 30.9% (n = 26) in other settings.

A statistically significant difference was also observed in experience related to the impact of immunosuppressive therapy on fertility among respondents working in primary care clinics, with lower levels of experience reported overall (p = 0.025). None of the respondents working in a primary care setting reported very high experience, compared to 20% (n = 20) in other settings.

No differences were found in the experience related to pregnancy-associated kidney diseases across workplace types, including multispecialty hospitals, district hospitals, specialist outpatient clinics, or private facilities. The summary of this data can be found in Table 3.

Table 3. The summary of the respondents' level of clinical experience in the management of patients with CKD across various specialties: 1 (very low experience), 2 (low experience), 3 (moderate experience), 4 (high experience), 5 (very high experience).

Question 1: Managing patients with CKD.					
	1	2	3	4	5
Number	10	5	17	16	68
Percentage	8.62%	4.31%	14.66%	13.79%	58.62%
Question 2: The impact of gender-related factors on the development of kidney diseases.					
	1	2	3	4	5
Number	23	27	23	23	20
Percentage	19.83%	23.28%	19.83%	19.83%	17.24%
Question 3: Kidney diseases related to pregnancy.					
	1	2	3	4	5
Number	39	27	26	17	7
Percentage	33.62%	23.28%	22.41%	14.66%	6.03%
Question 4: The impact of immunosuppressive therapy on fertility.					
	1	2	3	4	5
Number	32	19	26	19	20
Percentage	27.59%	16.38%	22.41%	16.38%	17.24%

3.1.3. Women's Health-Related Issues in Medical History

The survey revealed considerable variation in the frequency of collecting reproductive health-related information during medical history-taking. Most respondents reported routinely asking about menstrual regularity, with 41.3% (n = 48) doing so often and 19% (n = 22) always, while 32.8% (n = 38) asked rarely and only 6.9% (n = 8) never addressed this topic. Questions regarding pregnancy history were more consistently included, with 71.6% (n = 83) of physicians asking often or always. Similarly, 61.2% (n = 71) inquired about previous miscarriages with regularity, though nearly 40% (n = 45) did so infrequently or not at all. Perimenopausal symptoms were the least frequently addressed topic, with only 8.6% (n = 10) of respondents always asking and 19% (n = 22) never including this topic in routine assessments. Contraceptive use was discussed often or always by 65.4% (n = 77) of physicians, while 30.2% (n = 35) asked rarely. Questions about the timing of the last gynecological visit were common, with 74.7% (n = 89) asking often or always. Breast imaging (MMG/USG) and cervical cytology were also frequently addressed, with 65.5% (n = 76) and 68.1% (n = 79) of respondents, respectively, asking about these screenings regularly. The presented data is summarized in Figure 1.

https://doi.org/10.3390/jcm15010196

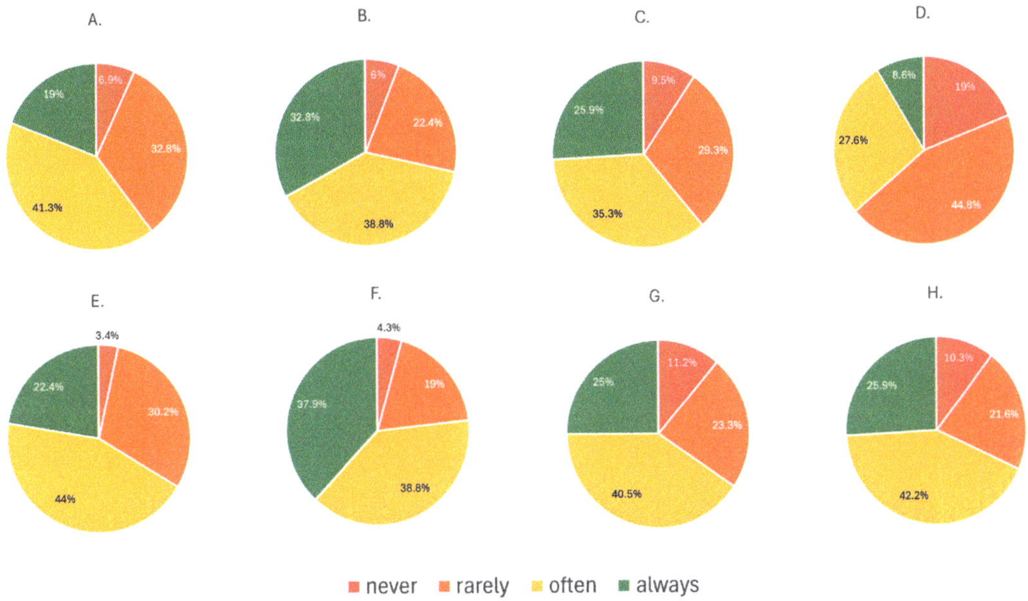

Figure 1. The summary of the responses regarding the frequency of addressing women's health issues while taking medical history: (**A**) menstrual regularity; (**B**) number of pregnancies; (**C**) number of miscarriages; (**D**) perimenopausal vasomotor symptoms; (**E**) use of contraception; (**F**) the date of the last gynecological visit; (**G**) the date of the last mammography (MMG) and breast ultrasound (USG); (**H**) the date of the last Pap-smear.

When asked about reproductive planning, 86.2% (n = 100) of physicians reported discussing procreative intentions with patients of reproductive age, although only half extended this question to both women and men. Most respondents (n = 77; 95.1%) with >10 years of experience reported routinely asking about reproductive plans, from which 51.9% (n = 42) asked only women, while 43.2% (n = 35) asked both women and men. However, 38.1% (n = 8) of respondents with <5 years of experience reported not asking such questions at all. This difference was statistically significant ($p < 0.001$).

In private healthcare facilities, 65.6% (n = 21) of respondents reported asking only women about reproductive plans, compared to 34.5% (n = 29) in other workplace settings. None of the respondents working in the private sector reported omitting this question entirely, while 19.1% (n = 16) of those practicing in other settings did. The association was statistically significant ($p < 0.001$).

A similar pattern was observed in specialist outpatient clinics, where 53.7% (n = 22) of respondents asked only women and only 2.4% (n = 1) omitted this question. This differed significantly from other settings ($p = 0.010$). In multispecialty hospitals, respondents were more likely to ask both women and men (46.4%, n = 39), while 16.7% (n = 14) did not ask at all ($p = 0.064$).

3.1.4. Survey Insights on Angiotensin-Converting Enzyme Inhibitors or Angiotensin II Receptor Blockers ACE-I/ARBs Use

Most respondents (n = 112, 96.6%) reported using ACE-I or ARBs in their clinical practice. Regardless of the number of years of clinical experience, the majority reported using this class of drugs: 95.2% (n = 20) with <5 years, 100.0% (n = 14) with 5–10 years, and 96.3% (n = 78) with >10 years. The difference between these groups was not found to be

https://doi.org/10.3390/jcm15010196

statistically significant. The use of ACE-I/ARB was also consistent between all workplace settings; the differences between various facilities were not significant.

These medications were most prescribed for either one or for more indications simultaneously, including hypertension (n = 110; 98.2%), nephroprotection (n = 104; 92.9%), and heart failure or cardioprotection (n = 98; 87.5%). Other indications were reported by 10.7% (n = 12) of physicians.

Reproductive health considerations were variably addressed when initiating ACE-I/ARB therapy. While 41.1% (n = 46) of respondents always asked about procreative plans prior to initiation of the treatment, 28.6% (n = 32) did so often, and 23.2% (n = 26) rarely. A small proportion (n = 8; 7.1%) never addressed this issue.

Nearly half of the physicians (n = 57; 50.9%) consistently informed patients about the important teratogenic risks associated with ACE-I/ARB use, while 24.1% (n = 27) did so frequently and 18.7% (n = 21) rarely. Similarly, 45.6% (n = 51) always discussed the need for contraception during treatment, though 30.3% (n = 34) did so infrequently or not at all.

Documentation of these discussions in medical records was inconsistent among respondents. Only 33% (n = 37) reported always recording and providing patients with the information about teratogenicity and contraception, while 36.6% (n = 41) did so rarely, and 16.1% (n = 18) never documented such details. The summary of the data can be found in Figure 2.

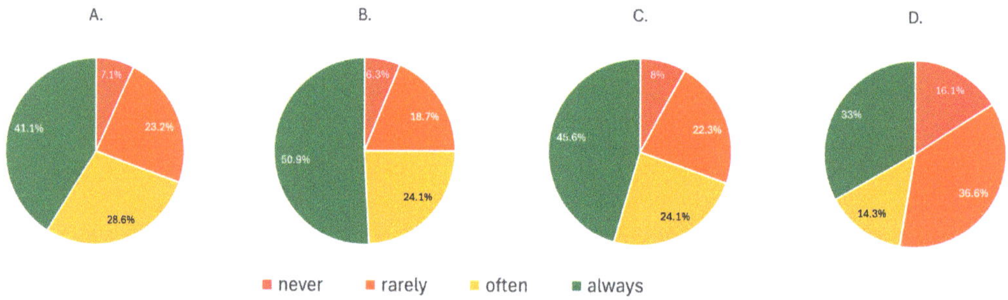

Figure 2. The summary of the responses regarding the frequency of addressing women's health issues during initiation of ACE-I/ARB therapy: (**A**) discussion about procreative plans of the patient; (**B**) information provided about teratogenic risks; (**C**) counseling on the need for contraceptive use during treatment; (**D**) documentation of teratogenic risk and contraceptive counseling in the medical record.

3.2. *Responses to Nephrologist-Specific Questions*

3.2.1. The Assessment of Focus on Women's Health-Related Issues During Residency Training

According to survey results, reproductive and sex-specific issues in nephrology are addressed inconsistently across residency programs. The influence of sex on the progression of kidney disease was addressed in a limited way according to the majority of respondents (n = 53, 66,2%), while 21.3% (n = 17) stated it was not covered at all. Similarly, the impact of CKD on fertility was also taught in a limited manner, as indicated by 66.3% of respondents (n = 52), with only 7.2% (n = 6) reporting comprehensive coverage.

Fertility of patients on dialysis was slightly better represented, with 36.2% (n = 29) of respondents indicating full coverage, although 56.3% (n = 45) still reported limited inclusion in the residency training. The broader topic of kidney disease and fertility followed a similar pattern, with 66.2% (n = 53) reporting partial coverage and only 25% (n = 20) full coverage.

https://doi.org/10.3390/jcm15010196

The impact of immunosuppressive therapy on fertility was the most thoroughly addressed topic, with over half of respondents (n = 41; 51.2%) reporting full coverage and 42.5% (n = 34) indicating limited inclusion.

Pregnancy-related nephrology topics were generally underrepresented. Management of pregnant women with CKD was covered in full according to only 20% (n = 16) of respondents, while 67.5% (n = 54) reported limited inclusion into the residency program. Unique aspects of dialysis during pregnancy were the least consistently taught topic, with nearly one in four respondents (n = 19, 23.8%) stating it was not covered at all, and only 18.7% (n = 15) reporting receiving comprehensive training. Similarly, kidney diseases specific to pregnancy were addressed in full according to just 25% (n = 20) of respondents, with 61.2% (n = 49) indicating limited coverage. The summary of the answers is gathered in Figure 3.

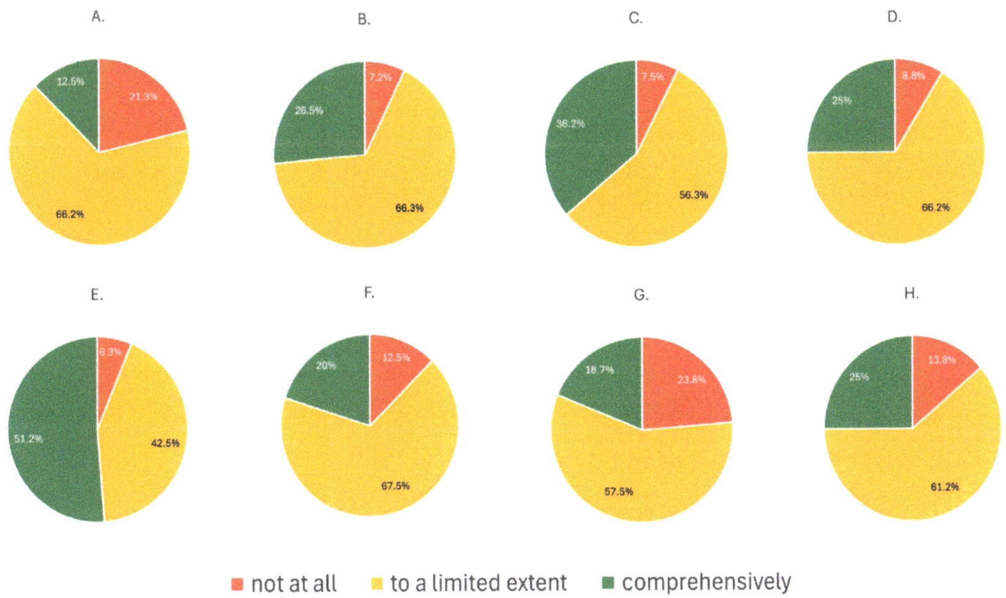

Figure 3. The summary of respondents' perceptions regarding the coverage of women's health topics during residency training: (**A**) the impact of gender-related factors on the progression of kidney diseases; (**B**) the impact of CKD on fertility; (**C**) the impact of dialysis on fertility; (**D**) the impact of kidney diseases on fertility; (**E**) the impact of immunosuppressive therapy on fertility; (**F**) the management of women with CKD during pregnancy; (**G**) dialysis during pregnancy; (**H**) kidney diseases specific to pregnancy.

3.2.2. Level of the Clinical Experience in the Management of Women's Health

Nephrology residents and specialists reported varying levels of clinical experience in managing sex-specific and reproductive aspects of CKD. In assessing sex-related differences in CKD progression, 8.8% (n = 7) rated their experience as minimal, 22.5% (n = 18) as low, 30% (n = 24) as moderate, 28.8% (n = 23) as high, and 10.0% (n = 8) as very high. In this field, 44.3% (n = 31) of specialists reported high or very high experience, compared to none among residents; among them, 80% (n = 8) reported minimal or low experience. This difference between these two groups was statistically significant ($p < 0.001$).

Regarding the selection of immunosuppressive therapy in patients of reproductive age, 11.3% (n = 9) reported minimal experience, 21.3% (n = 17) low, 16.3% (n = 13) moderate, 30.0% (n = 24) high, and 21.3% (n = 17) very high. The difference between specialists and

https://doi.org/10.3390/jcm15010196

residents was also significant in the level of experience in this field ($p = 0.024$), with 55.7% (n = 39) of specialists reporting high or very high experience, while 70% (n = 7) of residents reported minimal or low experience.

In the area of pregnancy planning for women with CKD, 6.3% (n = 5) reported minimal experience, 26.3% (n = 21) low, 26.3% (n = 21) moderate, 23.8% (n = 19) high, and 17.5% (n = 14) very high. It was rated as high or very high by 47.1% (n = 33) of specialists, compared to none among residents. Minimal or low experience was reported by 80% (n = 8) of residents ($p < 0.001$).

When asked about the impact of CKD on fertility, 7.5% (n = 6) reported minimal experience, 15% (n = 12) low, 31.3% (n = 25) moderate, 27.5% (n = 22) high, and 18.8% (n = 15) very high. Around half of specialists (51.4%; n = 36) have high or very high experience, compared to none among residents. Half of the residents (50%, n = 5) reported minimal experience ($p < 0.001$).

The lowest levels of experience both in the specialists and residents groups were reported in the area of assisted reproductive technologies (ART) in women with CKD, with 45% (n = 36) of all answers indicating minimal experience, 30% (n = 24) low, 15% (n = 12) moderate, and only 7.5% (n = 6) and 2.5% (n = 2) measured it as high and very high respectively. All residents (100%, n = 10) reported minimal experience, compared to 37.1% (n = 26) of specialists. Only 11.4% (n = 8) of specialists reported high or very high experience ($p = 0.001$). The summary of the data can be found in Table 4.

3.2.3. The Assessment of the Opinions on the Need to Implement More Women's Health-Related Issues into the Nephrology Care in Poland

Survey respondents expressed strong support for integrating sex-specific and reproductive health issues into nephrology care and residency training. A majority agreed that kidney disease therapy should be individualized based on patient sex, with 58.8% (n = 47) selecting "rather agree" and 32.5% (n = 26) "strongly agree" on this statement. Only 8.7% (n = 7) disagreed to any extent. The majority of residents (n = 9; 90%) and 90% (n = 63) of specialists agreed to the statement.

The need for establishing referral centers for pregnant women with CKD was affirmed by 58.8% (n = 47) who "strongly agreed" and 27.5% (n = 22) who "rather agreed," while only 13.7% (n = 11) expressed disagreement. There was no significant difference between residents and specialists on this (n = 8; 80% vs. n = 61; 87,1%).

Collaboration between gynecologists and nephrologists in the care of women with CKD was widely endorsed, with 86.3% (n = 69) "strongly agreeing" and 13.7% (n = 11) "rather agreeing" to the necessity of such cooperation. The 80% (n = 8) of residents and 87.1% (n = 61) of specialists strongly agreeing to the statement.

Regarding reproductive planning, 72.5% (n = 58) "strongly agreed" that renal replacement therapy should be adapted to patients' procreative intentions, and 25% (n = 20) "rather agreed." Only 2.5% (n = 2) disagreed, with 90% (n = 9) of residents and 70% (n = 49) of specialists strongly agreeing.

Similarly, 86.3% (n = 69) "strongly agreed", from which 90% (n = 9) of residents, and 85.7% (n = 60) of specialists, and 13.7% (n = 11) "rather agreed" that immunosuppressive treatment should be individualized based on reproductive plans.

In the multiple-choice question, among the 80 respondents who selected at least one answer, the most frequently selected form of training to gain more experience and knowledge on women's health and kidney diseases was the use of guidelines and recommendations from nephrology and gynecology societies, which was chosen by 72 doctors from this group. Conferences were also a preferred form chosen by 55 respondents, and webinars by 51. Additional specialist courses were selected by 42 participants, while 35 indicated

https://doi.org/10.3390/jcm15010196

mandatory specialist courses as a desirable format. The data regarding this question is summarized in Figures 4 and 5.

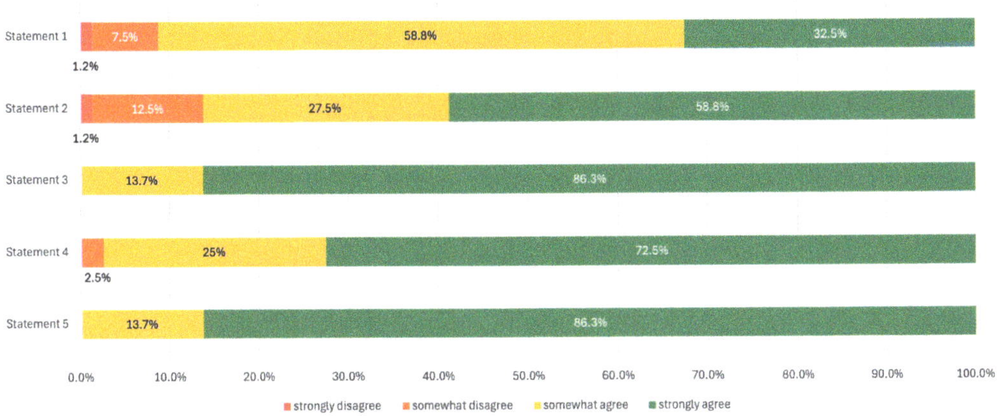

Figure 4. The assessment of the opinions on the need to implement more women's health-related issues into the nephrology care in Poland: **Statement 1**: It is essential to emphasize the necessity of tailoring kidney disease therapies based on the patient's gender. **Statement 2:** There is a need to establish reference centers for women with CKD during pregnancy. **Statement 3**: Close collaboration between gynecologists and nephrologists is essential in the management of patients with CKD. **Statement 4**: It is necessary to tailor the form of renal replacement therapy to the procreative plans of the patient. **Statement 5**: The individualization of immunosuppressive therapy in kidney diseases based on the patient's reproductive plans is essential.

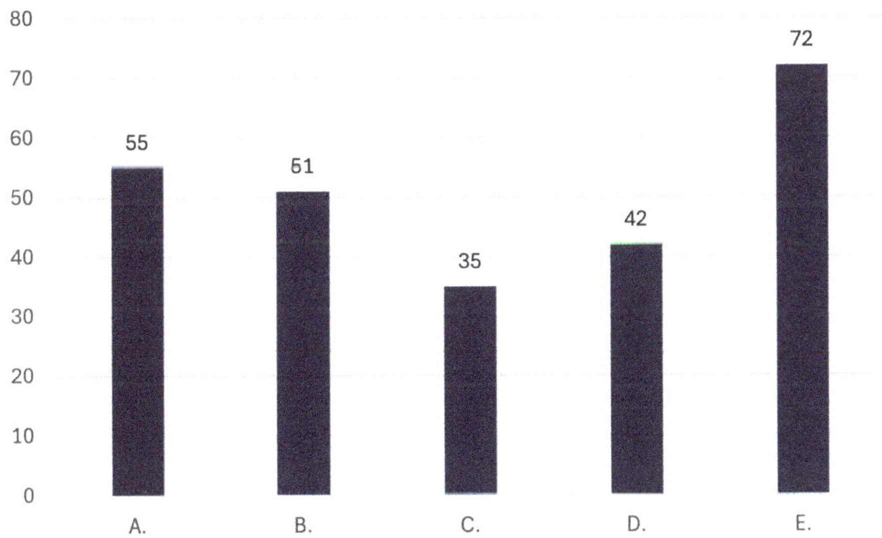

Figure 5. The summary of the preferred educational formats for advancing knowledge on women's health in kidney disorders (number of respondents): (**A**) conferences; (**B**) webinars; (**C**) mandatory courses during residency; (**D**) additional courses during residency; (**E**) guidelines and recommendations from nephrology and gynecology scientific societies.

https://doi.org/10.3390/jcm15010196

Table 4. Summary of the nephrologists' level of clinical experience in management of women's health: 1 (very low experience), 2 (low experience), 3 (moderate experience), 4 (high experience), 5 (very high experience).

Question 1: Differences in the course and progression of CKD based on the patient's gender.					
	1	2	3	4	5
Number	7	18	24	23	8
Percentage	8.75%	22.50%	30.00%	28.75%	10.00%
Question 2: Appropriate selection of immunosuppressive therapy for individuals of reproductive age.					
	1	2	3	4	5
Number	9	17	13	24	17
Percentage	11.25%	21.25%	16.25%	30.00%	21.25%
Question 3: Planning pregnancy in patients with CKD.					
	1	2	3	4	5
Number	5	21	21	19	14
Percentage	6.25%	26.25%	26.25%	23.75%	17.50%
Question 4: Differences in dialysis management during pregnancy.					
	1	2	3	4	5
Number	18	17	20	11	14
Percentage	22.50%	21.25%	25.00%	13.75%	17.50%
Question 5: The impact of CKD on fertility.					
	1	2	3	4	5
Number	6	12	25	22	15
Percentage	7.50%	15.00%	31.25%	27.50%	18.75%
Question 6: Assisted reproductive technologies (ART) in women with CKD.					
	1	2	3	4	5
Number	36	24	12	6	2
Percentage	45.00%	30.00%	15.00%	7.50%	2.50%

4. Discussion

The urgent need to incorporate women's health and reproductive issues into the management and treatment of patients with kidney disease has been recently extensively recognized and discussed by the Kidney Disease: Improving Global Outcomes (KDIGO) committee [10]. Our survey has followed similar ones performed in various populations of doctors around the world with the shared aim of trying to assess the level of knowledge and confidence among physicians in managing various sex-specific differences in kidney health [13–15].

Our results highlight the substantial burden of CKD among patients managed by specialists across various fields. Nearly all respondents (97.4%, n = 113) reported caring for individuals diagnosed with CKD. However, the true prevalence may be even higher, as demonstrated by a recent retrospective epidemiological study conducted in a primary care population. CKD was identified in 14.2% of patients from a high-risk group, based on either eGFR or urinary albumin-to-creatinine ratio (uACR) criteria [16]. These findings underscore the need for heightened diagnostic vigilance, particularly in primary care settings where early detection may be less systematic.

According to our study, the highest levels of self-reported experience in CKD management were observed among physicians working in private practices. In contrast, primary

https://doi.org/10.3390/jcm15010196

care practitioners generally rated their experience lower, especially regarding sex-specific factors in kidney disease. This observation is partially supported by findings from a Polish survey conducted by Jazienicka-Kiełb et al., which indicated that primary care physicians possess a solid foundational understanding of CKD management, yet expressed a strong interest in further education on the topic [17]. Expanding this educational scope to include sex- and gender-related aspects of kidney health, particularly those relevant to women's reproductive care, may be a valuable next step in strengthening primary care engagement with nephrology. The strong will of doctors to further expand their knowledge has also been demonstrated in our research.

As revealed in the survey, doctors do not consistently report data relevant to women's health, such as menstrual history, number of pregnancies, miscarriages, and contraception use. This has also been indicated in other studies conducted among nephrologists in the United States of America (USA) and Canada, which reported that doctors tend to omit taking and reporting a thorough obstetric history, which may lead to missing relevant data on patients' risk during pregnancy or for future kidney health [13]. However, doctors tend to address procreative plans issues mostly with women, while not always inquiring about these issues with male patients as stated by around 43% of respondents. Still, the common immunosuppressive drug—cyclophosphamide—remaining one of the most potent and commonly used therapeutic agents in the management of various glomerular disorders, poses a significant deleterious impact on both female and male fertility [18].

Another significant issue in the context of women's reproductive health concerns the use of ACE-I and ARBs. These medications play a well-established role in the management of both hypertension and CKD, as recommended by current clinical guidelines [19,20]. However, due to their known teratogenic effects, ACE-I/ARBs are contraindicated during pregnancy [21]. This presents a significant therapeutic challenge for physicians managing women with CKD who are planning pregnancy or are of childbearing age. Our study revealed that although physicians are generally aware of the risks associated with ACE-I/ARB use during pregnancy, the topic is often overlooked in clinical conversations. Specifically, many respondents reported that they do not routinely address the need for effective contraception when initiating these therapies in women of reproductive age. This gap in communication may reflect time constraints, assumptions about patient awareness, or discomfort discussing reproductive planning while managing patients with kidney disorders. The same conclusions come from the study conducted among the population of women aged 15–45 in the primary care in East London. 81,4% of patients with prescribed ACE-I/ARB had no previous preconception advice recorded [22].

The survey results indicated that both nephrology specialists and residents perceive their training programs as insufficient in preparing them to manage women's health issues in the context of kidney disorders. Topics related to fertility and pregnancy were reported to be addressed to a limited extent, which was expressed by most respondents. Although, women constitute the majority of patients with CKD [6], the prevalence among women of childbearing age tends to be relatively low—around 3% [23], birth rates in this population are significantly reduced (35.7 children per 1000 person years) compared to non-CKD individuals (46.5 children per 1000 person years) as observed in a population-based study conducted among women in the Stockholm region [24].

The level of expertise in managing female patients with CKD appears to correlate with years of clinical practice, as demonstrated by our survey results. This suggests that clinical confidence in addressing sex-specific aspects of nephrology care is largely acquired through hands-on experience rather than formal training. The limited exposure reported by residents and early-career professionals points to a gap in the current residency program, where topics related to women's reproductive health in CKD. Introducing these issues

https://doi.org/10.3390/jcm15010196

earlier in training may significantly enhance both confidence and perceived competence among future nephrologists. Especially, experience in pregnancy-related issues such as pregnancy planning and dialysis during pregnancy was reported to be low, even among specialists. Similar findings were reported in a survey conducted in Germany, where only 40% of nephrologists expressed confidence in managing pregnant patients undergoing dialysis. That study emphasized the urgent need for clearer, evidence-based guidelines to standardize care for pregnant women with CKD and to support clinicians in navigating these complex scenarios [15].

Women with CKD, especially those with already end-stage kidney disease (ESKD), experience various complex issues from hormonal imbalance [25] to sexual dysfunctions [26], which may impair their chances of conceiving naturally. In the event of progress of the assisted reproductive technologies (ART) methods, this procedure becomes a possible solution for this group of patients. Notably, the Italian Society of Nephrology has issued a best practice position statement regarding the various methods of medically associated reproduction. The study group has recognized ART methods as a possible option for women with CKD; however, their opinion is cautious, considering a potential increase in the risk of complications among these patients. The statement has called for personalized counselling with a multidisciplinary healthcare team [27]. To compare, most respondents in our survey have also agreed that a strong collaboration with gynecologists and creating reference centers should become a priority while addressing women's health in CKD.

It has been revealed in our study that nephrologists express a strong need for further education in the area of women's health within nephrology. The respondents consider guidelines either developed within nephrology or in collaboration with gynecological societies as a preferred way for addressing these topics and improving clinical competence. To our knowledge Polish Society of Nephrology working group has only addressed the issue of managing pregnancy in CKD; however, other related topics, such as preconception counselling, have not been covered yet. Such comprehensive practice guidelines have already been developed in the Netherlands [28], UK [29], Italy [27,30], or Germany [31].

Similar practice statements and guidelines have also been developed in other fields of medicine. The Working Group of the European Alliance of Associations for Rheumatology (EULAR) has also addressed the need for a clear consensus regarding the use of immunosuppressive medications in male patients and during pregnancy and lactation [32]. Selecting appropriate therapies during these critical periods is also a crucial consideration in the management of patients with glomerular diseases and renal manifestations of other autoimmune disorders. The teratogenic effects and reproductive risks associated with cancer treatment have been extensively discussed by oncology societies, which strongly advocate for comprehensive reproductive counseling. This includes the implementation of fertility preservation strategies such as embryo, oocyte, and ovarian tissue cryopreservation (OTC), ovarian transposition, and conservative gynecologic surgery [33,34]. These options should also be considered when initiating treatment with cyclophosphamide, a drug known for its detrimental impact on fertility. Concurrent administration of gonadotropin-releasing hormone agonists (GnRHa) may help preserve ovarian function and improve the likelihood of pregnancy in the future [35]. Given the growing engagement of the medical community in terms of reproductive health, this calls for an updated version of the Polish guidelines.

Our study obviously was not without limitations. Although it was not possible to determine the exact number of physicians who received the survey, the response rate was relatively low despite broad distribution across various workplace settings. This introduces the possibility of selection bias. The survey included both specialists, residents, and physicians from various fields; this heterogeneity may limit the specificity of conclusions for individual subgroups. However, this diversity reflects real-world clinical practice

https://doi.org/10.3390/jcm15010196

in Poland, where CKD care is delivered across multiple specialties and different levels of training.

Given the rising CKD and the limited number of nephrologists in Poland, a substantial proportion of patients, particularly those in early stages, are likely to be managed within primary care. Therefore, conducting a similar survey exclusively among primary care physicians would be valuable to more accurately assess their level of expertise and preparedness in addressing women's health issues in the context of CKD. Such data could inform targeted educational initiatives and promote earlier referral to nephrology services when appropriate [36].

The study mostly relied on self-reported measures of clinical experience using Likert scales. This approach is widely and commonly used in this type of research to assess the perceived level of competence and training needs. However, objective measures, including the exact number of CKD-pregnancy cases managed or the number of reproductive health issues addressed, could strengthen future studies; they were not feasible to collect due to the limited number of voluntary participants.

Despite these limitations, the study offers valuable insights into current practices and unmet educational needs in the management of sex-specific and reproductive health issues in CKD and highlights areas where targeted educational interventions and guideline development may be beneficial.

5. Conclusions

To conclude, our study has highlighted a critical discrepancy between the recognized importance of significant sex-specific and reproductive health considerations in the management of CKD and the current level of clinical experience and preparedness to implement these aspects in routine care. Although doctors generally agree on the need for more patient-centered, individualized care and interdisciplinary collaboration, the practical experience in managing female patients with complex issues such as pregnancy planning, renal-replacement therapies during pregnancy, and fertility-related care remains limited. Respondents expressed a clear willingness to obtain more educational tools on this topic. To ensure more equitable care for women with CKD, it seems pivotal to integrate reproductive health issues into nephrology training and develop interdisciplinary guidelines to ensure clear management pathways. By addressing current gaps in this field, it will be possible not only to improve clinical confidence among specialists but also advance the quality of care for a growing population of female patients whose needs for a long time have been unrecognized in nephrology.

Supplementary Materials: The following supporting information can be downloaded at: https://www.mdpi.com/article/10.3390/jcm15010196/s1.

Author Contributions: Conceptualization, W.P., A.R. and J.M.; methodology, W.P., K.G., A.R. and J.M.; software W.P. and K.G.; validation W.P., K.G., A.R. and J.M.; formal analysis W.P., A.R. and J.M.; investigation W.P. and B.B.; resources W.P., K.G. and B.B.; data curation W.P., K.G., B.B. and A.R.; writing—original draft preparation W.P. and B.B., writing—review and editing W.P., K.G., A.R. and J.M.; visualization, W.P. and K.G., supervision A.R. and J.M., funding acquisition J.M. All authors have read and agreed to the published version of the manuscript.

Funding: This research received no external funding.

Institutional Review Board Statement: The survey study was approved by the Ethics Committee of the Medical University of Warsaw (protocol code AKBE/94/2025, 17 March 2025).

Informed Consent Statement: All survey participants were informed of the anonymous collection of the data.

Data Availability Statement: The original contributions presented in this study are included in the article. Further inquiries can be directed to the corresponding author.

Acknowledgments: During the preparation of this study, the authors used Copilot, Microsoft, 365 for the purposes of data analysis and interpretation, and text editing and proofreading. The authors have reviewed and edited the output and take full responsibility for the content of this publication.

Conflicts of Interest: The authors declare no conflicts of interest.

Abbreviations

The following abbreviations are used in this manuscript:

ACE-I/ARBs	angiotensin-converting enzyme inhibitors or angiotensin II receptor blockers
ART	assisted reproductive technologies
CKD	chronic kidney disease
eGFR	estimated glomerular filtration rate
EULAR	European Alliance of Associations for Rheumatology
GnRHa	gonadotropin-releasing hormone agonists
HELIUS	Healthy Life in an Urban Setting
KDIGO	Kidney Disease: Improving Global Outcomes
MMG	mammography
NCD	noncommunicable disease
OTC	ovarian tissue cryopreservation
uACR	urinary albumin-to-creatinine ratio
USA	the United States of America
USG	ultrasound
WHO	World Health Organisation

References

1. Bikbov, B.; Purcell, C.A.; Levey, A.S.; Smith, M.; Abdoli, A.; Abebe, M.; Adebayo, O.M.; Afarideh, M.; Agarwal, S.K.; Agudelo-Botero, M.; et al. Global, Regional, and National Burden of Chronic Kidney Disease, 1990–2017: A Systematic Analysis for the Global Burden of Disease Study 2017. *Lancet* **2020**, *395*, 709–733. [CrossRef]
2. Reducing the Burden of Noncommunicable Diseases Through Promotion of Kidney Health and Strengthening Prevention and Control of Kidney Disease. Available online: https://apps.who.int/gb/ebwha/pdf_files/EB156/B156_CONF6-en.pdf (accessed on 1 September 2025).
3. Francis, A.; Harhay, M.N.; Ong, A.C.M.; Tummalapalli, S.L.; Ortiz, A.; Fogo, A.B.; Fliser, D.; Roy-Chaudhury, P.; Fontana, M.; Nangaku, M.; et al. Chronic Kidney Disease and the Global Public Health Agenda: An International Consensus. *Nat. Rev. Nephrol.* **2024**, *20*, 473–485. [CrossRef] [PubMed]
4. Lou-Meda, R.; Pérez, J.B. Reducing the Burden of Chronic Kidney Disease in the World. *Lancet* **2025**, *405*, 1810. [CrossRef]
5. Deng, L.; Guo, S.; Liu, Y.; Zhou, Y.; Liu, Y.; Zheng, X.; Yu, X.; Shuai, P. Global, Regional, and National Burden of Chronic Kidney Disease and Its Underlying Etiologies from 1990 to 2021: A Systematic Analysis for the Global Burden of Disease Study 2021. *BMC Public Health* **2025**, *25*, 636. [CrossRef]
6. Carrero, J.J.; Hecking, M.; Chesnaye, N.C.; Jager, K.J. Sex and Gender Disparities in the Epidemiology and Outcomes of Chronic Kidney Disease. *Nat. Rev. Nephrol.* **2018**, *14*, 151–164. [CrossRef]
7. Vosters, T.G.; Kingma, F.M.; Stel, V.S.; Jager, K.J.; van Ittersum, F.J.; van den Born, B.-J.H.; Vogt, L.; van Valkengoed, I.G.M. The Association and Contribution of Gender-Related Characteristics to Prevalent Chronic Kidney Disease in Women and Men in a Multi-Ethnic Population—The HELIUS Study. *BMC Public Health* **2025**, *25*, 853. [CrossRef]
8. Tong, A.; Evangelidis, N.; Kurnikowski, A.; Lewandowski, M.; Bretschneider, P.; Oberbauer, R.; Baumgart, A.; Scholes-Robertson, N.; Stamm, T.; Carrero, J.J.; et al. Nephrologists' Perspectives on Gender Disparities in CKD and Dialysis. *Kidney Int. Rep.* **2022**, *7*, 424–435. [CrossRef] [PubMed]
9. Prejbisz, A.; Dobrowolski, P.; Doroszko, A.; Olszanecka, A.; Tycińska, A.; Tykarski, A.; Adamczak, M.; Begier-Krasińska, B.; Chrostowska, M.; Dzida, G.; et al. Guidelines for the Management of Hypertension in Poland 2024—The Position of the Polish Society of Hypertension/Polish Cardiac Society Experts. *Arter. Hypertens.* **2024**, *28*, 91–146. [CrossRef]

https://doi.org/10.3390/jcm15010196

10. Piccoli, G.B.; Ahmed, S.B.; Fakhouri, F.; Garovic, V.D.; Hladunewich, M.A.; Jesudason, S.; Prakash, J.; Webster, A.C.; Zakharova, E.; Cheung, M.; et al. Women and Kidney Health: Conclusions from a Kidney Disease: Improving Global Outcomes (KDIGO) Controversies Conference. *Kidney Int.* **2025**, *108*, 355–379. [CrossRef] [PubMed]
11. Pinho-Gomes, A.-C.; Carcel, C.; Woodward, M.; Hockham, C. Women's Representation in Clinical Trials of Patients with Chronic Kidney Disease. *Clin. Kidney J.* **2023**, *16*, 1457–1464. [CrossRef]
12. Zucker, I.; Prendergast, B.J. Sex Differences in Pharmacokinetics Predict Adverse Drug Reactions in Women. *Biol. Sex Differ.* **2020**, *11*, 32. [CrossRef]
13. Hendren, E.M.; Reynolds, M.L.; Mariani, L.H.; Zee, J.; O'Shaughnessy, M.M.; Oliverio, A.L.; Moore, N.W.; Hill-Callahan, P.; Rizk, D.V.; Almanni, S.; et al. Confidence in Women's Health: A Cross Border Survey of Adult Nephrologists. *J. Clin. Med.* **2019**, *8*, 176. [CrossRef]
14. Ramesh, S.; James, M.T.; Holroyd-Leduc, J.M.; Wilton, S.B.; Seely, E.W.; Wheeler, D.C.; Ahmed, S.B. Sex Hormone Status in Women with Chronic Kidney Disease: Survey of Nephrologists' and Renal Allied Health Care Providers' Perceptions. *Can. J. Kidney Health Dis.* **2017**, *4*, 2054358117734534. [CrossRef]
15. Duffner, J.; Schulte-Kemna, L.; Reister, B.; Ludwig, U.; Keller, F.; Erp, R.V.; Schröppel, B. Survey among Nephrologists in Germany: Current Practice and Management of Pregnant Women on Dialysis. *Clin. Nephrol.* **2017**, *88*, 264–269. [CrossRef] [PubMed]
16. Jazienicka, A.; Babicki, M.; Krajewska, M.; Oko, A.; Kłoda, K.; Biesiada, A.; Mastalerz-Migas, A. A Nationwide Epidemiological Study of Chronic Kidney Disease Prevalence in a High-Risk Patient Population Without Prior Diagnosis in Primary Health Care in Poland. *J. Clin. Med.* **2025**, *14*, 3600. [CrossRef]
17. Jazienicka-Kiełb, A.; Babicki, M.; Krajewska, M.; Oko, A.; Kłoda, K.; Mastalerz-Migas, A. Assessment of Primary Care Physicians' Knowledge of Chronic Kidney Disease in Poland. *Front. Public Health* **2022**, *10*, 1032240. [CrossRef] [PubMed]
18. Perez-Garcia, L.F.; Dolhain, R.J.E.M.; Vorstenbosch, S.; Bramer, W.; Van Puijenbroek, E.; Hazes, J.M.W.; Te Winkel, B. The Effect of Paternal Exposure to Immunosuppressive Drugs on Sexual Function, Reproductive Hormones, Fertility, Pregnancy and Offspring Outcomes: A Systematic Review. *Hum. Reprod. Update* **2020**, *26*, 961–1001. [CrossRef]
19. Stevens, P.E.; Ahmed, S.B.; Carrero, J.J.; Foster, B.; Francis, A.; Hall, R.K.; Herrington, W.G.; Hill, G.; Inker, L.A.; Kazancıoğlu, R.; et al. KDIGO 2024 Clinical Practice Guideline for the Evaluation and Management of Chronic Kidney Disease. *Kidney Int.* **2024**, *105*, S117–S314. [CrossRef]
20. McEvoy, J.W.; McCarthy, C.P.; Bruno, R.M.; Brouwers, S.; Canavan, M.D.; Ceconi, C.; Christodorescu, R.M.; Daskalopoulou, S.S.; Ferro, C.J.; Gerdts, E.; et al. 2024 ESC Guidelines for the Management of Elevated Blood Pressure and Hypertension. *Eur. Heart J.* **2024**, *45*, 3912–4018. [CrossRef] [PubMed]
21. Countouris, M.; Mahmoud, Z.; Cohen, J.B.; Crousillat, D.; Hameed, A.B.; Harrington, C.M.; Hauspurg, A.; Honigberg, M.C.; Lewey, J.; Lindley, K.; et al. Hypertension in Pregnancy and Postpartum: Current Standards and Opportunities to Improve Care. *Circulation* **2025**, *151*, 490–507. [CrossRef]
22. Lovegrove, E.; Robson, J.; McGettigan, P. Pregnancy Protection and Pregnancies in Women Prescribed ACE Inhibitors or ARBs: A Cross-Sectional Study in Primary Care. *Br. J. Gen. Pract.* **2020**, *70*, e778–e784. [CrossRef]
23. Webster, P.; Lightstone, L.; McKay, D.B.; Josephson, M.A. Pregnancy in Chronic Kidney Disease and Kidney Transplantation. *Kidney Int.* **2017**, *91*, 1047–1056. [CrossRef]
24. Vrijlandt, W.A.L.; De Jong, M.F.C.; Prins, J.R.; Bramham, K.; Vrijlandt, P.J.W.S.; Janse, R.J.; Mazhar, F.; Carrero, J.J. Prevalence of Chronic Kidney Disease in Women of Reproductive Age and Observed Birth Rates. *J. Nephrol.* **2023**, *36*, 1341–1347. [CrossRef]
25. Rojas, R.; Clegg, D.J.; Palmer, B.F. Amenorrhea and Estrogen Disorders in Kidney Disease. *Semin. Nephrol.* **2021**, *41*, 126–132. [CrossRef]
26. Pyrgidis, N.; Mykoniatis, I.; Tishukov, M.; Sokolakis, I.; Nigdelis, M.P.; Sountoulides, P.; Hatzichristodoulou, G.; Hatzichristou, D. Sexual Dysfunction in Women with End-Stage Renal Disease: A Systematic Review and Meta-Analysis. *J. Sex. Med.* **2021**, *18*, 936–945. [CrossRef]
27. Attini, R.; Cabiddu, G.; Ciabatti, F.; Montersino, B.; Carosso, A.R.; Gernone, G.; Gammaro, L.; Moroni, G.; Torreggiani, M.; Masturzo, B.; et al. Chronic Kidney Disease, Female Infertility, and Medically Assisted Reproduction: A Best Practice Position Statement by the Kidney and Pregnancy Group of the Italian Society of Nephrology. *J. Nephrol.* **2023**, *36*, 1239–1255. [CrossRef]
28. De Jong, M.F.C.; Van Hamersvelt, H.W.; Van Empel, I.W.H.; Nijkamp, E.J.W.; Lely, A.T. Summary of the Dutch Practice Guideline on Pregnancy Wish and Pregnancy in CKD. *Kidney Int. Rep.* **2022**, *7*, 2575–2588. [CrossRef] [PubMed]
29. Wiles, K.; Chappell, L.; Clark, K.; Elman, L.; Hall, M.; Lightstone, L.; Mohamed, G.; Mukherjee, D.; Nelson-Piercy, C.; Webster, P.; et al. Clinical Practice Guideline on Pregnancy and Renal Disease. *BMC Nephrol.* **2019**, *20*, 401. [CrossRef]
30. Cabiddu, G.; Spotti, D.; Gernone, G.; Santoro, D.; Moroni, G.; Gregorini, G.; Giacchino, F.; Attini, R.; Limardo, M.; Gammaro, L.; et al. A Best-Practice Position Statement on Pregnancy after Kidney Transplantation: Focusing on the Unsolved Questions. The Kidney and Pregnancy Study Group of the Italian Society of Nephrology. *J. Nephrol.* **2018**, *31*, 665–681. [CrossRef] [PubMed]

https://doi.org/10.3390/jcm15010196

31. Schmidt, M.; Stracke, S.; Schneider, U.; Kuschel, B.; Feldkamp, T.; Habbig, S.; Mayer-Pickel, K.; Hartung, A.; Bader, B.; Weinmann-Menke, J.; et al. Chronic Kidney Disease and Pregnancy. Guideline of the DGGG, OEGGG, DGfN (S2k Level, AWMF Registry No. 015–090). *Geburtshilfe Frauenheilkd* **2022**, *82*, 795–830. [CrossRef] [PubMed]
32. Rüegg, L.; Pluma, A.; Hamroun, S.; Cecchi, I.; Perez-Garcia, L.F.; Anderson, P.O.; Andreoli, L.; Wirström, S.B.; Boyadhzieva, V.; Chambers, C.; et al. EULAR Recommendations for Use of Antirheumatic Drugs in Reproduction, Pregnancy, and Lactation: 2024 Update. *Ann. Rheum. Dis.* **2025**, *84*, 910–926. [CrossRef] [PubMed]
33. Lambertini, M.; Peccatori, F.A.; Demeestere, I.; Amant, F.; Wyns, C.; Stukenborg, J.-B.; Paluch-Shimon, S.; Halaska, M.J.; Uzan, C.; Meissner, J.; et al. Fertility Preservation and Post-Treatment Pregnancies in Post-Pubertal Cancer Patients: ESMO Clinical Practice Guidelines. *Ann. Oncol.* **2020**, *31*, 1664–1678. [CrossRef] [PubMed]
34. Su, H.I.; Lacchetti, C.; Letourneau, J.; Partridge, A.H.; Qamar, R.; Quinn, G.P.; Reinecke, J.; Smith, J.F.; Tesch, M.; Wallace, W.H.; et al. Fertility Preservation in People with Cancer: ASCO Guideline Update. *J. Clin. Oncol.* **2025**, *43*, 1488–1515. [CrossRef] [PubMed]
35. Ejaz, K.; Abid, D.; Juneau, P.; Chu, J.; Hasni, S. Use of Gonadotropin-Releasing Hormone Agonists for Ovarian Preservation in Patients Receiving Cyclophosphamide for Systemic Lupus Erythematosus: A Meta-Analysis. *Lupus* **2022**, *31*, 1706–1713. [CrossRef]
36. Srialluri, N.; Thavarajah, S. CKD in Reproductive-Aged Women: A Call for Early Nephrology Referral and Multidisciplinary Care. *BMC Nephrol.* **2024**, *25*, 444. [CrossRef]

https://doi.org/10.3390/jcm15010196

Journal of
Clinical Medicine

MDPI

Article

Beyond Dialysis Adequacy: Transportation Time and Pain as Quality-of-Life Predictors in Polish Hemodialysis Patients—A Single-Center Study

Stanisław Rączewski [1,2,†], Weronika Caban [1,2,†], Natalia Lemiszewska [1,2], Mikołaj Kuncewicz [1,2], Magdalena Mosakowska [1], Ewa Kotwica-Strzałek [1,3,*] and Stanisław Niemczyk [1]

1 Department of Internal Medicine, Nephrology and Dialysis, Military Institute of Medicine-National Research Institute, 04-141 Warsaw, Poland; sniemczyk@wim.mil.pl (S.N.)
2 Faculty of Medicine, Medical University of Warsaw, 02-091 Warsaw, Poland
3 Department of Descriptive and Clinical Anatomy, Medical University of Warsaw, 02-004 Warsaw, Poland
* Correspondence: ekotwica@wim.mil.pl
† These authors contributed equally to this work.

Abstract

Background: Dialysis adequacy (Kt/V) remains an essential marker of hemodialysis quality; however, it does not fully capture patients' overall well-being. Growing evidence underscores the need for a more holistic, patient-centered approach that integrates clinical efficiency with factors affecting daily functioning and quality of life (QoL). **Objectives:** This study aimed to identify the key determinants of health-related quality of life (HRQoL) among Polish patients undergoing hemodialysis. **Methods:** Seventy hemodialysis patients from a single center completed the KDQOL-36 questionnaire and provided demographic and clinical data. Statistical analyses included Pearson's and Spearman's correlations, as well as multiple linear regression, to determine predictors of HRQoL. **Results:** The mean (SD) KDQOL summary score was 60.9 (17.3). Pain ($B = -15.9$, $p < 0.001$) and the need for additional dialysis sessions ($B = -10.2$, $p = 0.008$) were the strongest independent predictors of poorer HRQoL, collectively accounting for 28.6% of variance. Longer dialysis-related transportation time ($r = -0.238$, $p = 0.03$) and longer hemodialysis vintage ($r = -0.254$, $p = 0.03$) were also significantly associated with lower HRQoL, while dialysis adequacy showed no significant effect. **Conclusions:** Pain, additional dialysis sessions, and longer dialysis-related transportation time are key, modifiable contributors to reduced HRQoL in Polish hemodialysis patients. These findings underscore the importance of a patient-centered approach that supplements clinical measures with interventions targeting comfort, education, and accessibility. Incorporating structured pain management and improved transport into routine nephrology practice can meaningfully improve patient QoL.

Keywords: chronic kidney disease; hemodialysis; pain; quality of life; commute burden

1. Introduction

Health-related quality of life (HRQoL) is a crucial outcome measure in hemodialysis (HD) patients, as it is associated with mortality, hospitalization, and overall patient well-being [1]. The Kidney Disease Quality of Life Short Form (KDQOL-36) is one of the most widely validated instruments for measuring QoL in dialysis populations, demonstrating reliability across multiple domains [2,3]. Analysis of patient responses yields scores in five domains: physical component summary, mental component summary, burden of kidney disease, symptoms and problems associated with kidney disease, and effects of kidney disease [2].

Previous studies have demonstrated an association between HRQoL and disease management [1,4]. Common factors associated with lower QoL among chronic kidney disease patients include older age, lower education, poverty, and social dysfunction. Additionally, pain and non-adherence to dietary restrictions have been recognized as significant barriers to patient well-being; however, their relative importance compared to biochemical adequacy remains unclear. Current trends in nephrology suggest that the need for supplemental dialysis should be minimized through robust educational efforts. The occurrence of extra sessions often results from both patient-related factors, such as non-adherence to dietary and fluid restrictions, and clinical management challenges within the dialysis process itself [5].

Kt/V is an index used to quantify dialysis adequacy, calculated by comparing pre- and post-dialysis blood urea nitrogen levels. For decades, Kt/V has been a central component of dialysis adequacy guidelines. Current KDOQI guidelines recommend a minimum single-pool Kt/V of approximately 1.2 per dialysis session for thrice-weekly hemodialysis to ensure adequate waste removal [6].

This study aimed to identify which clinical and organizational factors most strongly influence HRQoL among HD patients. The examined variables included sociodemographic characteristics, dialysis adequacy, dialysis vintage, duration of each dialysis session, and a summary of dialysis-related transportation time to and from the dialysis center, including waiting time for medical transport after dialysis sessions, number of hospitalizations, and perceived pain.

While quality of life has been studied globally, there is a lack of recent data focusing on the specific logistical and clinical challenges within the Polish healthcare system. By identifying the impact of transportation time and pain in a representative urban cohort, this study aims to provide actionable insights for improving patient-centered care at the institutional and regional levels.

2. Materials and Methods

A single-center, cross-sectional analytical study was conducted at the Dialysis Unit of the Department of Internal Medicine, Nephrology and Dialysotherapy at the Military Institute of Medicine—National Research Institute in Warsaw, Poland. The center serves the general civilian population as a tertiary care public hospital. The study group included adult patients undergoing maintenance hemodialysis, representative of the general population of hemodialysis patients in Poland

The study was approved by an institutional medical ethics committee at the Military Institute of Medicine—National Research Institute in Warsaw, Poland (decision number 34/25, 25 June 2025). All participants provided written informed consent to participate in the study. All patient personal details were anonymized and kept confidential throughout the analysis and reporting process.

The study cohort consisted of 70 hemodialysis patients who consented to participation and met the inclusion criteria, as follows: (1) age $\geq$ 18 years, (2) undergoing maintenance hemodialysis, and (3) clinical stability. Patients with acute illness, severe cognitive impairment, or inability to complete questionnaires were excluded. Participants completed the KDQOL-36 questionnaire and a demographic survey that included age, gender, education level, marital status, employment status, necessity of additional dialysis in last 6 months, and etiology of kidney disease. Additional clinical data were collected, including previous hospitalizations (within the past 6 months), dialysis frequency (in sessions per week), and commute time to and from the dialysis center, including waiting time for organized medical transportation. For the exploratory analysis of the study population, patients were stratified into two subgroups based on their health-related quality of life outcomes. The required criterion for this split was the mean KDQOL summary score calculated for the entire cohort (60.91 points). Patients achieving a score above this threshold were categorized into the 'Higher QoL' group, while those below were assigned to the 'Lower QoL' group.

In the KDQOL-36 questionnaire, each subscale score ranges from 0 to 100, with higher scores indicating better HRQoL. Thus, a higher score reflects fewer symptoms, lower perceived burden, or better physical and mental well-being, depending on the subscale. In contrast, lower scores indicate greater symptom severity, higher disease burden, or poorer functioning in the respective domains.

The questionnaire was administered either through face-to-face interviews or as self-administered questionnaires, depending on the patient's preference. Participants were informed that they could decline to answer any question or withdraw from the study at any time. All responses were collected during dialysis sessions at the facility. All patient data were anonymized immediately after collection and assigned identification numbers for data analysis.

Descriptive statistics, including means, standard deviations, and frequencies, were calculated for all variables. Before statistical analysis, the normality of KDQOL values was confirmed using the Shapiro–Wilk test. For bivariate associations, Pearson's and Spearman's correlation coefficients were used for normally distributed continuous variables, and Spearman's rho for non-parametric data. Independent samples t-tests compared group means (additional dialysis vs. no additional dialysis; pain present vs. absent), while chi-square tests evaluated associations between categorical variables. To identify independent predictors of KDQOL scores, multiple linear regression analysis was performed, entering all significant univariate variables. Statistical significance was set at $p < 0.05$. The strength r—Pearson correlation coefficient. was interpreted as follows: $|r| < 0.3$—weak; $0.3 \leq |r| < 0.5$—moderate; $|r| \geq 0.5$—strong relationship. Positive values indicate a direct correlation, while negative values indicate an inverse relationship. All analyses were conducted using IBM SPSS version 29 Statistical software.

3. Results

3.1. Sociodemographic Characteristics

Sociodemographic characteristics are summarized in Table 1. The total number of patients included in the study cohort was 70. The patients' ages ranged from 36 to 90 years, with a mean of 68.24 years (SD = 11.08 years). The majority of participants were male, at 61.4%. A total of 28 individuals (40.0%) were married. Most participants were not working, with 58 (82.9%) mostly retired and 46 (65.7%) retired. The predominant level of education completed was secondary, with 44 (62.9%) individuals. To further explore the data, the study population was divided into two subgroups based on the mean KDQOL summary score (60.91 points). The first group consisted of 34 patients (48.6%) with scores above the mean (KDQOL > Mean), representing better health-related quality of life, while the second group included 36 patients (51.4%) with scores below the mean (KDQOL < Mean). No significant differences in age or gender distribution were observed between the groups, although a trend toward lower quality of life was noted in older patients.

3.2. Clinical Characteristics

Clinical characteristics of the study population are summarized in Table 2. The most common cause of kidney disease was chronic kidney disease associated with diabetes, being the leading cause among 19 (27.1%) participants. All patients underwent scheduled hemodialysis sessions three times per week, with the mean (SD) dialysis duration of 3.48

(0.40) hours. The mean (SD) single-pool Kt/V obtained in our study group was 1.17 (0.24), which is below the minimal value of 1.2 and target dose of 1.4 recommended by the KDIGO guidelines. The mean (SD) of HD vintage was 45.36 (40.60) months. During the previous 6 months, 38.6% of patients required at least one additional dialysis session, and 58.6% were hospitalized, with a mean (SD) hospitalization duration of 11.14 (18.74) days.

Table 1. Sociodemographic characteristics of the study population.

Variable	Female	Male	KDQOL > Mean	KDQOL < Mean	All (%)
Age group (years)	**27 (38.6)**	**43 (61.4)**	**34 (48.6)**	**36 (51.4)**	70
<65	6 (22.2)	13 (30.0)	11 (32.4)	8 (22.2)	19 (27.1)
≥65	21 (77.8)	30 (70.0)	23 (67.6)	28 (77.8)	59 (84.3)
Marital Status					
Married	6 (22.2)	22 (51.2)	14 (41.1)	14 (38.8)	28 (40.0)
Single	4 (14.8)	7 (16.3)	7 (20.6)	4 (11.1)	11 (15.7)
Widowed	13 (48.1)	8 (18.6)	10 (29.4)	11 (30.5)	21 (30.0)
Divorced	4 (14.8)	6 (13.9)	3 (8.8)	7 (19.4)	10 (14.3)
Occupation					
Employed	6 (22.2)	6 (13.9)	5 (14.7)	7 (19.4)	12 (17.1)
Unemployed	1 (3.7)	2 (4.7)	2 (5.9)	1 (2.7)	3 (4.3)
Retired	19 (70.4)	27 (62.8)	22 (64.7)	24 (66.7)	46 (65.7)
Medical pension	1 (3.7)	8 (18.6)	5 (14.7)	4 (11.1)	9 (12.9)
Educational status					
Primary	2 (7.4)	3 (7.0)	2 (5.9)	3 (8.3)	5 (7.1)
Secondary	17 (63.0)	27 (62.8)	21 (61.8)	23 (63.9)	44 (62.9)
Tertiary	8 (29.6)	13 (30.2)	11 (32.3)	10 (27.8)	21 (30.0)

Showing number of patients (percentage).

Table 2. Clinical characteristics of the study population.

Variable	Frequency (%)	Mean (SD)
Dialysis per week		3.00 (0)
Vintage (months of HD)		45.36 (40.60)
Dialysis duration (hours)		3.48 (0.40)
Kt/V		1.17 (0.24)
Commute time (hours) [1]		4.89 (2.77)
Additional dialyses		
Yes	27 (38.6)	
No	43 (61.4)	
Hospitalization (last 6 months)		
Yes	41 (58.6)	11.14 (18.74) days
No	29 (41.4)	
Experienced pain		
Yes	42 (60.0)	
No	28 (40.0)	
Etiology of kidney disease		
Chronic kidney disease associated with diabetes	19 (27.1)	
Hypertensive nephropathy	2 (2.9)	
Obstructive uropathy	7 (10.0)	
Polycystic kidney disease	7 (10.0)	
Unclear	18 (25.7)	
Other	17 (24.3)	

[1] Total commute time-including the wait for organized medical transport; SD, Standard Deviation; HD, Hemodialysis.

https://doi.org/10.3390/jcm15041423

3.3. Baseline QoL Characteristics

Quality of Life Characteristics, based on the five KDQOL-36 subscales and two summary scores, are shown in Table 3. The highest mean score was observed on the Symptoms and Problems subscale (74.97), indicating that, on average, patients reported relatively few symptoms or concerns. While the Burden of Kidney Disease subscale had the lowest mean score (44.1), indicating a higher perceived burden of the disease among patients, it also showed the broadest score range (SD of 30.43).

Table 3. Baseline characteristics, $n = 70$.

Component	Mean	SD
Summary KDQOL score	60.91	17.33
Symptoms and problems	74.97	16.47
Effects of the kidney disease	65.63	19.86
Burden of the kidney disease	44.10	30.43
SF-12 Physical health composite	35.28	11.47
SF-12 Mental health composite	49.03	11.58

Scores range from 0 to 100, where higher values indicate better health-related quality of life.

3.4. Correlation Between Sociodemographic and Clinical Data

3.4.1. Sociodemographic Variables and Clinical Parameters

Sociodemographic variables, such as age (B = −0.06, $p = 0.72$), sex (B = −1.32, $p = 0.73$), education (B = 3.57, $p = 0.26$), and marital status (B = 1.39, $p = 0.39$), did not show significant associations with the KDQOL scores.

Experiencing pain was negatively correlated with all KDQOL subscales, indicating a strong negative association with quality of life across all domains.

Hemodialysis vintage was negatively correlated with SF-12 Physical component scores ($p = 0.03$), meaning that a longer duration of HD treatment was associated with lower physical health scores. No significant correlations were observed between hemodialysis vintage and KDQOL subscale scores. Similarly, Kt/V values showed no significant correlation with any of the assessed quality-of-life measures. The values are presented in Table 4.

Table 4. Correlation between quality of life and dialysis parameters.

Variable	Vintage of HD	Kt/V Value	Pain
KDQOL	−0.187	−0.039	**−0.524** *
Symptoms and problems	−0.186	−0.001	**−0.493** *
Effects of the kidney disease	−0.07	−0.014	**−0.246** *
Burden of the kidney disease	−0.116	−0.034	**−0.305** *
SF-12 Physical	**−0.254** *	−0.014	**−0.340** *
SF-12 Mental	0.021	−0.07	**−0.729** *

r values from Pearson's and Spearman's correlations; statistically significant correlations ($p < 0.05$) are shown in bold and marked with *.

3.4.2. Need for Additional Dialysis Sessions

Patients requiring additional dialysis had significantly lower KDQOL scores in all KDQOL subscales ($p < 0.05$), except for the SF-12 mental health composite. A comparison of mean KDQOL subscale scores is presented in Table 5. The results indicate poorer physical health and a greater disease burden among patients requiring additional dialysis. The lack of a significant difference found in the SF-12 mental health composite (t = 0.789, $p = 0.22$) suggests that the groups have comparable mental health statuses.

https://doi.org/10.3390/jcm15041423

Table 5. Comparison of KDQOL mean scores based on the need for additional dialysis.

Additional Dialyses	*n*	KDQOL	Symptoms and Problems	Effects of the Kidney Disease	Burden of the Kidney Disease	SF-12 Physical	SF-12 Mental
Required	27	**53.73** *	**70.66** *	**56.83** *	**34.49** *	**27.58** *	47.70
Not required	43	**65.42** *	**77.66** *	**71.15** *	**50.15** *	**35.23** *	49.95

Statistically significant correlations ($p < 0.05$) are shown in bold and marked with *; means compared using Student's t test; Scores range from 0 to 100, where higher values indicate better health-related quality of life.

3.4.3. Total Dialysis Transportation Burden, Dialysis Duration

Comparison between commute and dialysis times is shown in Table 6. Longer dialysis-related transportation time (including waiting for organized medical transport) to the hemodialysis site was significantly associated with lower scores on the effects of kidney disease subscale (r = −0.258; $p = 0.047$) and the general KDQOL score (r = −0.238; $p = 0.03$). Dialysis session duration showed no significant association with any of the subscales.

Table 6. Correlation of HRQoL with commute and dialysis durations.

Variable	Mean (SD)	KDQOL	Symptoms and Problems	Effects of the Kidney Disease	Burden of the Kidney Disease	SF-12 Physical	SF-12 Mental
Commute time [1]	4.89 (2.77)	**−0.258** *	−0.139	**−0.238** *	−0.150	−0.205	−0.110
Dialysis time	3.48 (0.40)	−0.160	−0.188	−0.210	−0.058	−0.131	0.021

[1] Total commute time, including the wait for organized medical transport; SD, Standard Deviation r values from Pearson's and Spearman's correlations; statistically significant correlations ($p < 0.05$) are shown in bold and marked with *.

3.4.4. Regression Analysis

Prior to multivariable modeling, univariate linear regression analyses were performed to examine the crude associations between each candidate predictor and KDQOL total score. Variables considered included age, sex, educational level, marital status. Variables showing a univariate association with KDQOL at $p < 0.20$, as well as variables considered clinically relevant based on prior literature, were retained for multivariable analysis.

A multiple linear regression model was then constructed to identify independent predictors of KDQOL while adjusting for potential confounders. KDQOL total score was treated as the dependent variable, and age, sex, educational level, marital status, additional dialysis sessions, and pain experience were entered simultaneously as independent variables. These covariates were selected a priori due to their plausible associations with quality of life in patients undergoing dialysis.

The overall model was statistically significant ($F(6, 63) = 5.604$, $p < 0.001$), indicating that the included predictors collectively explained a significant proportion of the variance in KDQOL scores. The adjusted coefficient of determination (adjusted $R^2 = 0.286$) suggested that approximately 28.6% of the variability in KDQOL was explained by the model, which is considered acceptable in observational studies of quality-of-life outcomes. Model assumptions, including linearity, homoscedasticity, normality of residuals, and absence of multicollinearity, were assessed and found to be acceptable.

After adjustment, pain experience (B = −15.93, $p < 0.001$) and additional dialysis sessions (B = −10.18, $p = 0.008$) were independently associated with lower KDQOL scores. Specifically, patients reporting pain had, on average, a 15.9-point lower KDQOL score compared with those without pain, while patients requiring additional dialysis sessions had a 10.2-point lower KDQOL score. Other covariates were not significantly associated with KDQOL in the multivariable model.

https://doi.org/10.3390/jcm15041423

4. Discussion

Our patients' demographic and treatment characteristics align with those observed in international HD populations assessed with the KDQOL-36 (Table 1) [4], except for markedly higher summary commute time. Our cohort demonstrates poor physical HRQoL and moderate kidney-disease-specific quality of life (Table 3), consistent with reports from the United States [3] and Polish populations [7]. Notably, the Symptoms and Problems subscale showed the highest scores. In contrast, the Burden of Kidney Disease subscale showed the lowest scores, indicating that patients experience a significant disease burden despite relatively few reported symptoms, which is consistent with previous studies.

Pain represents one of the most prevalent yet under-treated symptoms among patients with chronic kidney disease, with systematic review evidence demonstrating that approximately 60% of patients undergoing hemodialysis experience pain, significantly exceeding the 20% prevalence in the general population [5,8]. Our finding, that pain emerged as the strongest independent predictor of reduced health-related quality of life among all subscales ($B = -15.9$, $p < 0.001$) and explained substantial variance in HRQoL, aligns with this evidence and highlights the profound impact of pain on patient well-being. Patients undergoing hemodialysis face multiple pain sources, including procedure-related discomfort from repeated vascular access punctures, muscle cramps during or after dialysis sessions, and pain from prolonged sitting during treatments. Beyond dialysis-specific pain, many patients experience chronic musculoskeletal pain- the most common pain type in hemodialysis populations, affecting approximately 45% of patients. Musculoskeletal pain is often associated with mineral and bone disorders that accompany chronic kidney disease, which disrupt calcium and phosphorus homeostasis and increase the risk of fractures. Neuropathic pain, present in approximately 10% of patients, includes diabetic peripheral neuropathy among patients with chronic kidney disease associated with diabetes (27.1% in our cohort) and uremic neuropathy. These diverse pain sources create a complex situation where conventional analgesic approaches often fail to alleviate the pain adequately. Despite this high burden, pain remains systematically under-treated in dialysis populations, mainly due to limited awareness among healthcare providers and concerns about analgesic safety in patients with impaired kidney function [9,10]. Our results, showing that 60% of patients experienced pain and that pain was negatively correlated with all KDQOL-36 subscales, underscore the urgent need for comprehensive pain assessment and management strategies integrated into routine dialysis care. Evidence-based interventions should address multiple pain mechanisms, including optimizing vascular access techniques to minimize puncture-related pain, implementing intradialytic positioning protocols to reduce musculoskeletal discomfort, ensuring adequate management of bone mineral metabolism, and providing appropriate pharmacological treatment tailored to individual renal function. For neuropathic pain, which systematic review evidence identified as significantly associated with diabetes, hypertension, and higher BMI [8], specific agents such as gabapentin may be indicated, though dosing requires careful adjustment. Non-pharmacological approaches, including physical therapy, heat application for muscle cramps, and cognitive-behavioral interventions, also warrant consideration [8,10,11]. Given that pain was the single strongest predictor of quality of life in our cohort. Healthcare systems should prioritize systematic pain screening using validated tools, multidisciplinary pain management protocols, and staff education on pain recognition and treatment. Such comprehensive pain management strategies represent a critical yet underutilized opportunity to improve outcomes for hemodialysis patients significantly.

The negative correlation between longer duration of HD treatment and lower physical health scores may result from aging and the progression of underlying disease, leading to a

https://doi.org/10.3390/jcm15041423

decline in general condition commonly observed among elderly patients undergoing HD. However, this is not associated with increased mortality in this group [6,12].

The mere duration of the HD session was not associated with quality of life, which may be attributed to very similar dialysis times for most participants. Moreover, longer dialysis sessions have been associated with better survival and intermediate outcomes. Still, they may negatively impact social well-being, suggesting a complex relationship between the length of HD sessions and quality of life [13,14].

Dialysis adequacy in our cohort generally meets the minimal targets, with a mean single-pool Kt/V of 1.17. However, other cohorts achieve higher average Kt/V values, ranging from 1.4 to 1.5 [6,15]. We found no effect of dialysis adequacy on quality of life, and the absence of correlation underscores the limitations of depending exclusively on biochemical markers. This underscores the need to identify additional significant variables to enable more personalized care. An important observation in this study was that patients requiring additional dialysis sessions demonstrated significantly lower quality of life compared with those treated exclusively on a standard thrice-weekly schedule. This reduction was reflected in both the overall KDQOL summary score and in nearly all subscales. Although this may be partially explained by factors such as a higher uremic burden, greater comorbidity load, or inadequate clearance, it is most likely caused by non-adherence to fluid intake or dietary recommendations, leading to fluid overload and a subsequent need for extra dialysis. Implementing a structured educational process could address these gaps, reducing the need for treatment intensification and improving overall patient outcomes. Given that non-compliance with dietary and fluid guidelines is common among HD patients, the necessity of additional dialysis sessions should alert clinicians' attention [4,6,16]. Non-compliance results in a lower quality of life, a higher risk of hospitalizations, adverse outcomes, and even death, making it especially important to personalize care and recommendations and motivate patients accordingly. Additionally, the negative association between additional dialysis sessions and KDQOL suggests that either the factors leading to additional dialysis or increased dialysis burden may contribute to lower patient well-being. Interventions in this area could significantly improve adherence to restrictions, but they should include a cognitive or cognitive/behavioral component [1,4,17].

Dietetic support plays a pivotal role in enhancing adherence to dietary and fluid intake restrictions among HD patients. Non-adherence to these restrictions is prevalent, with studies indicating rates as high as 60%, which can lead to adverse health outcomes [18]. Engagement with dietetics professionals has been shown to address this issue effectively. For instance, structured nutrition education programs have demonstrated significant improvements in patients' adherence to dietary and fluid restrictions, as evidenced by reductions in interdialytic weight gain and improved blood pressure control [19].

Recent qualitative research from Spain further underscores the importance of dietitian involvement. Patients report that consistent, culturally sensitive guidance from dietitians empowers them to manage their dietary restrictions more effectively, resulting in improved health outcomes. Furthermore, caregivers recognize the support of renal dietitians as a crucial facilitator in assisting patients to adhere to dietary recommendations [11].

Incorporating dietetics professionals into the multidisciplinary care team is crucial for developing individualized dietary plans that account for patients' cultural and personal preferences. Such tailored interventions improve adherence and patients' quality of life by reducing the burden of dietary restrictions. The systematic review also suggests including cognitive or cognitive-behavioral components in such interventions [17].

Therefore, healthcare systems should prioritize integrating dietetic services into routine HD care to optimize patient outcomes. In the context of the Polish healthcare system, this underscores the need to integrate dietitian services into primary care for patients on hemodialysis. Such integration would enhance adherence to dietary and fluid intake recommendations, thereby improving patient outcomes.

4.1. Clinical Dialysis-Related Transportation Time

A longer combined commute and wait time to the dialysis site was significantly associated with lower HRQoL. This result is consistent with extensive international studies, which found that longer travel times were associated with a higher adjusted relative risk (RR) of death and worse HRQoL in HD patients across multiple subscales, even after adjusting for other factors [20,21]. Our findings regarding transportation time are particularly relevant in the context of the Polish healthcare infrastructure, suggesting that logistical improvements could be as impactful as clinical interventions in enhancing patient well-being. The negative impact of a long commute can be attributed to several causes. Foremost, transportation itself is time-consuming, effectively adding on to the "dialysis day" and reducing time for rest, family, or work [22]. It may also limit social activities and cause additional fatigue, pain (if transportation is uncomfortable), and stress. At least some patients in this HD station rely on ambulance transportation to our dialysis station, which may be associated with longer waiting and commute times due to inefficient transport, for example, waiting for other patients to complete dialysis. Consequently, even the patients who live close to the dialysis center, if they have reduced mobility, have to rely on group, time-consuming, and often delayed transport.

In various countries, alternatives to ambulance transport for HD patients have been implemented. For example, in multiple municipalities in the United States of America, patients may use private cars, taxis, or wheelchair-accessible vehicles to travel between their residences and healthcare facilities. Permission for such transport is granted based on medical assessments, and patients can receive reimbursement for these journeys [23].

The problem could also be improved by increasing the availability of home HD. Currently, in Denmark, home HD accounts for 7% of all dialysis treatments. It is mainly delivered using dialysis machines installed at no cost in patients' homes. Patients typically begin as limited-care in-center HD patients and transition to home hemodialysis after 3–6 months of training. Some centers in Denmark have adopted a "Home HD First" policy, resulting in higher home hemodialysis adoption rates (up to 14% in these centers). The policy emphasizes autonomy, improved outcomes, and cost-effectiveness. Additionally, Denmark has one of the highest rates of home dialysis in Europe, with 28% of patients treated at home, 21% with peritoneal dialysis, and 7% with home hemodialysis [24].

4.2. Limitations

There are several significant limitations to our findings. Most data were self-reported, sometimes via a single, non-validated question. Secondly, there could be substantial nonresponse bias. Non-responders were usually older, possibly feeling worse during HD, and therefore not keen to participate in the survey. Thirdly, this study was conducted at a single center, limiting the generalizability of the findings. Furthermore, the cross-sectional, single-time-point design of the study precludes the assessment of changes over time and does not allow for causal inferences regarding the identified predictors. Although the mean dialysis adequacy (Kt/V) in our study population did not meet the target threshold recommended by KDIGO guidelines, we did not observe a significant impact of this parameter on the reported quality of life outcomes or other primary findings. Our study did not include a formal nutritional assessment or sarcopenia evaluation. Furthermore, our study did not analyze the specific reasons for supplementary dialysis sessions or the extent of patient education, which are critical for optimizing the treatment process and avoiding unnecessary dialysis intensification. Validation in a multi-center setting is warranted.

https://doi.org/10.3390/jcm15041423

5. Conclusions

These results underscore the need for a more personalized, holistic model of dialysis care that balances clinical efficacy with patient comfort, access to services, and quality of life. In the context of Polish nephrology, particular attention should be paid to improving pain control, facilitating dietary adherence, and reducing logistical barriers to treatment. Further studies are needed regarding how individually tailored education programs, standardized pain management plans, and transportation support can be effectively integrated into routine, patient-centered dialysis care. Future research should focus on longitudinal assessments to track QoL dynamics and intervention-based studies evaluating the impact of dedicated transportation services and structured nutritional support. Furthermore, multicenter cohorts are warranted to confirm these findings on a national scale.

Author Contributions: Conceptualization, S.R. and W.C.; Methodology, S.R., W.C., N.L., M.K., M.M., E.K.-S. and S.N.; Formal analysis, W.C. and M.K.; Investigation, S.R., W.C., N.L., M.K., M.M. and E.K.-S.; Writing—original draft preparation, S.R., W.C., N.L. and M.K.; Writing—review and editing, S.R. and S.N.; Supervision, M.M., E.K.-S. and S.N. All authors have read and agreed to the published version of the manuscript.

Funding: This research received no external funding.

Institutional Review Board Statement: The study was conducted in accordance with the Declaration of Helsinki and approved by the Institutional Medical Ethics Committee at the Military Institute of Medicine—National Research Institute in Warsaw, Poland (decision number 34/25, 25 June 2025).

Informed Consent Statement: Informed consent was obtained from all subjects involved in the study.

Data Availability Statement: The data presented in this study are available on request from the corresponding author. The data are not publicly available due to privacy and ethical restrictions, as they contain information that could compromise the anonymity of the research participants.

Conflicts of Interest: The authors declare no conflicts of interest.

Abbreviations

The following abbreviations are used in this manuscript:

BMI	Body Mass Index
CKD	Chronic Kidney Disease
HD	Hemodialysis
HRQoL	Health-Related Quality of Life
KDOQI	Kidney Disease Outcomes Quality Initiative
KDQOL	Kidney Disease Quality of Life
Kt/V	Dialysis Adequacy Index
QoL	Quality of Life
RR	Relative Risk
SD	Standard Deviation
SF-12	Short Form 12 Health Survey
SPSS	Statistical Package for the Social Sciences

References

1. Durán-Gómez, N.; Martín Parrilla, M.; Montanero-Fernández, J.; López-Jurado, C.F.; Pérez-Civantos, D.; Cáceres León, M.C. Impact of mental health status and clinical factors on health-related quality of life in patients undergoing haemodialysis: A multicentre cross-sectional study. *BMJ Open* **2025**, *15*, e097506. [CrossRef]
2. Rao, S.; Carter, W.B.; Mapes, D.L.; Kallich, J.D.; Kamberg, C.J.; Spritzer, K.L.; Hays, R.D. Development of subscales from the symptoms/problems and effects of kidney disease scales of the kidney disease quality of life instrument. *Clin. Ther.* **2000**, *22*, 1099–1111. [CrossRef] [PubMed]

https://doi.org/10.3390/jcm15041423

3. Cohen, D.E.; Lee, A.; Sibbel, S.; Benner, D.; Brunelli, S.M.; Tentori, F. Use of the KDQOL-36™ for assessment of health-related quality of life among dialysis patients in the United States. *BMC Nephrol.* **2019**, *20*, 112. [CrossRef]
4. Speyer, E.; Tu, C.; Zee, J.; Sesso, R.; Lopes, A.A.; Moutard, E.; Omorou, A.Y.; Stengel, B.; Finkelstein, F.O.; Pecoits-Filho, R.; et al. Symptom Burden and Its Impact on Quality of Life in Patients With Moderate to Severe CKD: The International Chronic Kidney Disease Outcomes and Practice Patterns Study (CKDopps). *Am. J. Kidney Dis.* **2024**, *84*, 696–707.e691. [CrossRef] [PubMed]
5. Fletcher, B.R.; Damery, S.; Aiyegbusi, O.L.; Anderson, N.; Calvert, M.; Cockwell, P.; Ferguson, J.; Horton, M.; Paap, M.C.S.; Sidey-Gibbons, C.; et al. Symptom burden and health-related quality of life in chronic kidney disease: A global systematic review and meta-analysis. *PLoS Med.* **2022**, *19*, e1003954. [CrossRef]
6. Daugirdas, J.T.; Depner, T.A.; Inrig, J.; Mehrotra, R.; Rocco, M.V.; Suri, R.S.; Weiner, D.E.; Greer, N.; Ishani, A.; MacDonald, R.; et al. KDOQI Clinical Practice Guideline for Hemodialysis Adequacy: 2015 Update. *Am. J. Kidney Dis.* **2015**, *66*, 884–930. [CrossRef] [PubMed]
7. Dąbrowska-Bender, M.; Dykowska, G.; Żuk, W.; Milewska, M.; Staniszewska, A. The impact on quality of life of dialysis patients with renal insufficiency. *Patient Prefer. Adherence* **2018**, *12*, 577–583. [CrossRef]
8. Lambourg, E.; Colvin, L.; Guthrie, G.; Murugan, K.; Lim, M.; Walker, H.; Boon, G.; Bell, S. The prevalence of pain among patients with chronic kidney disease using systematic review and meta-analysis. *Kidney Int.* **2021**, *100*, 636–649. [CrossRef]
9. Davison, S.N.; Rathwell, S.; Ghosh, S.; George, C.; Pfister, T.; Dennett, L. The Prevalence and Severity of Chronic Pain in Patients With Chronic Kidney Disease: A Systematic Review and Meta-Analysis. *Can. J. Kidney Health Dis.* **2021**, *8*, 2054358121993995. [CrossRef]
10. Dember, L.M.; Hsu, J.Y.; Mehrotra, R.; Cavanaugh, K.L.; Kalim, S.; Charytan, D.M.; Fischer, M.J.; Jhamb, M.; Johansen, K.L.; Becker, W.C.; et al. Pain Coping Skills Training for Patients Receiving Hemodialysis. *JAMA Intern. Med.* **2025**, *185*, 197. [CrossRef]
11. Padial, M.; Avesani, C.M.; García-Testal, A.; Cana-Poyatos, A.; Lindholm, B.; Segura-Ortí, E. Dietary Needs, Barriers, and Facilitators Among Patients on Hemodialysis and Their Caregivers: The GoodRENal Project in Spain. *J. Ren. Nutr.* **2025**, *35*, 337–343. [CrossRef] [PubMed]
12. Yeung, E.K.; Brown, L.; Kairaitis, L.; Krishnasamy, R.; Light, C.; See, E.; Semple, D.; Polkinghorne, K.R.; Toussaint, N.D.; MacGinley, R.; et al. Impact of haemodialysis hours on outcomes in older patients. *Nephrology* **2023**, *28*, 109–118. [CrossRef]
13. Sułkowski, L.; Matyja, A.; Matyja, M. Social Support and Quality of Life in Hemodialysis Patients: A Comparative Study with Healthy Controls. *Medicina* **2024**, *60*, 1732. [CrossRef]
14. Ishiwatari, A.; Yamamoto, S.; Fukuma, S.; Hasegawa, T.; Wakai, S.; Nangaku, M. Changes in Quality of Life in Older Hemodialysis Patients: A Cohort Study on Dialysis Outcomes and Practice Patterns. *Am. J. Nephrol.* **2020**, *51*, 650–658. [CrossRef]
15. Robinson, B.M.; Akizawa, T.; Jager, K.J.; Kerr, P.G.; Saran, R.; Pisoni, R.L. Factors affecting outcomes in patients reaching end-stage kidney disease worldwide: Differences in access to renal replacement therapy, modality use, and haemodialysis practices. *Lancet* **2016**, *388*, 294–306. [CrossRef]
16. Lindberg, M.; Prütz, K.G.; Lindberg, P.; Wikström, B. Interdialytic weight gain and ultrafiltration rate in hemodialysis: Lessons about fluid adherence from a national registry of clinical practice. *Hemodial. Int.* **2009**, *13*, 181–188. [CrossRef]
17. Ekholm, M.; Aulbach, M.; Walsh, S.; Phipps, D.; Rauta, V.; Knittle, K. Behavioral interventions targeting treatment adherence in chronic kidney disease: A systematic review and meta analysis. *Soc. Sci. Med.* **2025**, *366*, 117594. [CrossRef]
18. Vr, V.; Kaur Kang, H. The Worldwide Prevalence of Nonadherence to Diet and Fluid Restrictions Among Hemodialysis Patients: A Systematic Review and Meta-analysis. *J. Ren. Nutr.* **2022**, *32*, 658–669. [CrossRef] [PubMed]
19. Başer, E.; Mollaoğlu, M. The effect of a hemodialysis patient education program on fluid control and dietary compliance. *Hemodial. Int.* **2019**, *23*, 392–401. [CrossRef] [PubMed]
20. Moist, L.M.; Bragg-Gresham, J.L.; Pisoni, R.L.; Saran, R.; Akiba, T.; Jacobson, S.H.; Fukuhara, S.; Mapes, D.L.; Rayner, H.C.; Saito, A.; et al. Travel time to dialysis as a predictor of health-related quality of life, adherence, and mortality: The Dialysis Outcomes and Practice Patterns Study (DOPPS). *Am. J. Kidney Dis.* **2008**, *51*, 641–650. [CrossRef]
21. Namimi-Halevi, C.; Keinan-Boker, L.; Dichtiar, R.; Beckerman, P.; Bromberg, M. Travel Distance to Dialysis and Mortality Among Hemodialysis Patients in a Geographically Small Country. *J. Community Health* **2025**, *50*, 1115–1126. [CrossRef] [PubMed]
22. Scholes-Robertson, N.J.; Howell, M.; Gutman, T.; Baumgart, A.; Sinka, V.; Tunnicliffe, D.J.; May, S.; Chalmers, R.; Craig, J.; Tong, A. Patients' and caregivers' perspectives on access to kidney replacement therapy in rural communities: Systematic review of qualitative studies. *BMJ Open* **2020**, *10*, e037529. [CrossRef]
23. Tian, F.F.; Hall, Y.N.; Griffin, S.; Kranze, T.; Marcella, D.; Watnick, S.; O'Hare, A.M. The Complex Patchwork of Transportation for In-Center Hemodialysis. *J. Am. Soc. Nephrol.* **2023**, *34*, 1621–1627. [CrossRef] [PubMed]
24. Heaf, J. The Danish Nephrology Registry. *Clin. Epidemiol.* **2016**, *8*, 621–627. [CrossRef] [PubMed]

https://doi.org/10.3390/jcm15041423

MDPI AG
Grosspeteranlage 5
4052 Basel
Switzerland
Tel.: +41 61 683 77 34

Journal of Clinical Medicine Editorial Office
E-mail: jcm@mdpi.com
www.mdpi.com/journal/jcm

www.ingramcontent.com/pod-product-compliance
Lightning Source LLC
Chambersburg PA
CBHW062101220926
51850CB00010B/2846
* 9 7 8 3 7 2 5 8 7 4 9 2 7 *